Dados Internacionais de Catalogação na Publicação (CIP)
(Câmara Brasileira do Livro, SP, Brasil)

Terassini, Flávio Aparecido
The fantastic world of parasites [livro eletrônico] : small, dangerous, and fascinating / Flávio Aparecido Terassini. -- Porto Velho, RO : Ed. do Autor, 2025.
PDF

Bibliografia.
ISBN 978-65-01-54823-4

1. Medicina e saúde 2. Parasitas 3. Parasitologia 4. Zoonoses I. Título.

25-281422 CDD-574.5249

Índices para catálogo sistemático:

1. Parasitologia : Biologia 574.5249

Eliane de Freitas Leite - Bibliotecária - CRB 8/8415

This is a work of nonfiction. While every effort has been made to ensure the accuracy of the information presented, this book is not intended to serve as medical advice. Readers are encouraged to consult qualified healthcare professionals regarding any medical concerns or before acting on any of the information provided.

Author: Flávio Aparecido Terassini
Title: The Fantastic World of Parasites: Small, Dangerous, and Fascinating
Language: English
ISBN: 9786501548234
Published Independently by the Author
Cover Design and Layout: Flávio Aparecido Terassini
First Edition – 2025

Cover image: *Upper arthropods: Assassin bug, Bed bug, Ticks, Flea, Mosquito and Cockroach.*
On the wing of the bat feeding on blood: *Larva of an Argasid tick feeding on a bat's wing.*
Photos by: *Flávio Aparecido Terassini.*

To my family, wife Mariana, my children Malu, Olívia and Tadeu, friends, mentors, colleagues, all those fascinated by the hidden world of parasites, and...

...also for the Wari Indigenous,
in January 2000, an Indigenous man from the Wari' village in Sagarana, on the Guaporé River in Guajará-Mirim, Rondônia, Brazil, called me:

"Uta Ixicum Coteca Trama Catim."

which translates to:

"I am the little and great Tick Man."

Words from my mentors

I can say that Flávio A. Terasini, who´s nickname is "Micuim", has been my friend and student since de 1998. He started working with me in 1999 in a project that aimed to describe the ticks fauna from Rondônia. He travelled a lot of times with me around Rondônia, capturing ticks for our research projects. For me, he is still a "kid", like a son. Very honest, dedicated to his work and a great enthusiast of science. I really admire he as an human being and a scientist. As we use to say in Brazil " I good soul".

By Luís Marcelo Aranha Camargo Ph.D

Researcher – Institute of Biomedical Sciences (ICB5 - USP) Monte Negro, Rondônia Brasil

When I first introduced ticks to Flavio A. Terassini in the year 2000, he was only 17 years old. One year later, at 18 years old, he was able to provide taxonomic identification of all ticks from the Brazilian fauna. Inevitably, in the intervening years he has found several new species of tick in the Brazilian Amazon, some of which we have officially described and others which are on the way. Today, Flavio is much more than a 'ticksman'; his contributions to the advancement of knowledge meet the diversity of the biome, which is grateful for all his good deeds as a great promoter and defender of the richest biome on the planet.

By Marcelo Bahia Labruna Ph.D

Researcher – University of São Paulo (USP), São Paulo, SP, Brazil

I have known Flavio A. Terrassini for a long time and have always admired him for his perseverance. Many people say they work hard, but few actually do. The battle is always hard in pursuit of your goals.

By Pedro Ismael da Silva Júnior Ph.D

Researcher – Butantan Institute - São Paulo, SP, Brazil

I met Flávio A. Terassini in Porto Velho as soon as I moved to Rondônia, back in 2015. At the time, I was pursuing my PhD and sought him out for guidance on ticks in Rondônia, and there I could realize his notable knowledge, passion for ticks, and sensitivity to nature. Life's circumstances led us to switch roles, on paper, and today, as an advisor, I'm being a kind of a professor-student, drinking from the experience of the TicksMan. Flávio has an acute intuition for the nature around him, and when combined with his teaching talent, it makes him a transformative force in Amazonian society and a true guardian of the Amazon rainforest.

By André de Abreu Rangel Aguirre, Ph.D.

Researcher – Fiocruz Rondônia, Porto Velho, RO, Brazil

Acknowledgment

First and foremost, I thank God for the gift of life, my family, my health, and the countless opportunities that have shaped my journey.

To my beloved parents, Antônio and Dirce, who, from an early age, taught me through their example to always strive to be my best—kind, attentive, and dedicated in everything I do. They instilled in me the importance of education, perseverance, and never giving up on my dreams and goals.

To my wife, my companion in all aspects of life, and the wonderful mother of our children—Malu, Olívia, and Tadeu—thank you for the beautiful and joyful family we share every day.

To my sister, Francielly, and my dear friends and mentors—Saymon, who graciously wrote the preface for this book, Kayena and Kaynara, Smith, and all my friends who, together, make this world a better place.

To my students from São Lucas Porto Velho-AFYA, Classe A, Maple Bear, and my online students from Hotmart—you will always hold a special place in my heart.

I extend my heartfelt gratitude to the Institute of Biomedical Sciences 5 (ICB5) at the University of São Paulo (USP), where my journey into scientific research began back in 1999. That initial opportunity ignited a lifelong passion for parasitology and the natural world.

I am also deeply thankful to the Instituto Butantan, where I had the privilege to continue learning and growing in 2002, immersed in a world-class environment of scientific excellence.

To Faculdade São Lucas-AFYA, I offer sincere thanks for providing me with the foundation of knowledge I have today and for the incredible opportunity to serve as a university professor. Since 2006, I have had the honor of teaching Parasitology, Tropical Diseases, and Research and Extension Projects to future medical professionals—an experience that fills me with pride and purpose every day.

I also express my gratitude to Fiocruz Rondônia, for welcoming me into its academic and scientific community as a PhD candidate, allowing me to continue evolving as a researcher and educator.

To those who inspire bold and creative science communication, I thank the team from Brave Wilderness—Mark, Mario, and Coyote Peterson—for being constant sources of motivation with their passion for the wild. A special thanks to Richard Rasmussen, whose partnership and commitment to wildlife education have enriched my mission. And finally, my appreciation to Mr. Lee Cockerell for his books, which offer uniquely inspiring insights into leadership, excellence, and purposeful living.

Thank you—truly, thank you all!

and first tip for ***Parasite Hunters:*** *Read every word in this book, from cover to back cover.*

Preface

You've probably watched—or at least heard of—the film *Alien, the Eighth Passenger* © 1979 Brandywine Productions. Distributed by 20th Century Fox. This 1979 science fiction masterpiece, brilliantly directed by Ridley Scott, was not only a massive box office and critical success, but also left audiences worldwide astonished by the story of a parasitic alien lifeform that used humans as hosts to complete its life cycle. The idea of a creature silently nesting inside another living being, feeding off its resources, and replicating, sparked both horror and—strangely—fascination.

Alien is just one of many stories with a similar theme: a disturbing creature, alien or not, that depends on another organism to survive, grow, and reproduce. What many fail to realize, however, is that this concept isn't just the stuff of fiction. It is a biological reality—startling, complex, often lethal—and it happens far closer than we might like to imagine (yes, perhaps even inside you, right now, as you read this).

In the most remote and forgotten corners of the planet, there are examples even more unsettling than what we see on screen. From the eye of a child in an African village, to the intestine of a peaceful missionary, the foot of a Southeast Asian farmer, or the liver of an Indigenous person in South America—parasites, invisible at first, take hold, feed, reproduce, and often profoundly alter the health and lives of their hosts.

In many developing countries, parasites remain one of the leading causes of public health crises. They affect entire local economies in areas with poor or no sanitation, diminish the quality of life for millions, and take lives silently. Even in developed countries, they haven't vanished—they've just become more discreet, though still present.

It is within this complex, fascinating, and at times, shadowy reality that we find Flávio Aparecido Terassini. Naturally curious, hyperactive, a tireless researcher—and above all—a passionate naturalist, Flávio has dedicated much of his life to exploring the world of parasites: their cycles, their strategies, their secrets.

With a career shaped by long stretches in the jungle, working with isolated riverine and Indigenous communities, traveling muddy roads, and peering through stereoscopic magnifiers, he has explored Brazil's many biomes—especially the vast, mysterious Amazon Rainforest.

Flávio is one of those rare scientists who combines technical precision with a deep, almost poetic wonder for nature. His eyes are trained (almost supernaturally so) to notice what others overlook. He remembers names, taxonomic changes, and host relationships with an enviable memory and sharp intuition.

He has led and participated in dozens of scientific expeditions, mentored research, and uncovered organisms previously unknown to science. Talking to him about parasites feels like listening to a master storyteller—except these stories aren't myths; they're astonishing realities.

And now, with the generosity of someone who truly knows his craft, Flávio offers us this book. More than just a scientific guide, it's a deep dive into a world as invisible as it is essential. With clear, engaging language—without ever sacrificing scientific accuracy—he takes us on a journey through the winding paths of parasitology, revealing the complexity, the beauty, and the brutality of these organisms that share our planet (even when we wish they didn't).

Get ready for a journey of discovery—and prepare to be amazed. Because after reading this book, you'll never see nature the same way again.

By Saymon de Albuquerque, Ph.D.

Biologist, Professor and Researcher – São Lucas, Porto Velho, RO – AFYA

Summary

Chapter 1

Parasite Hunter Challenge

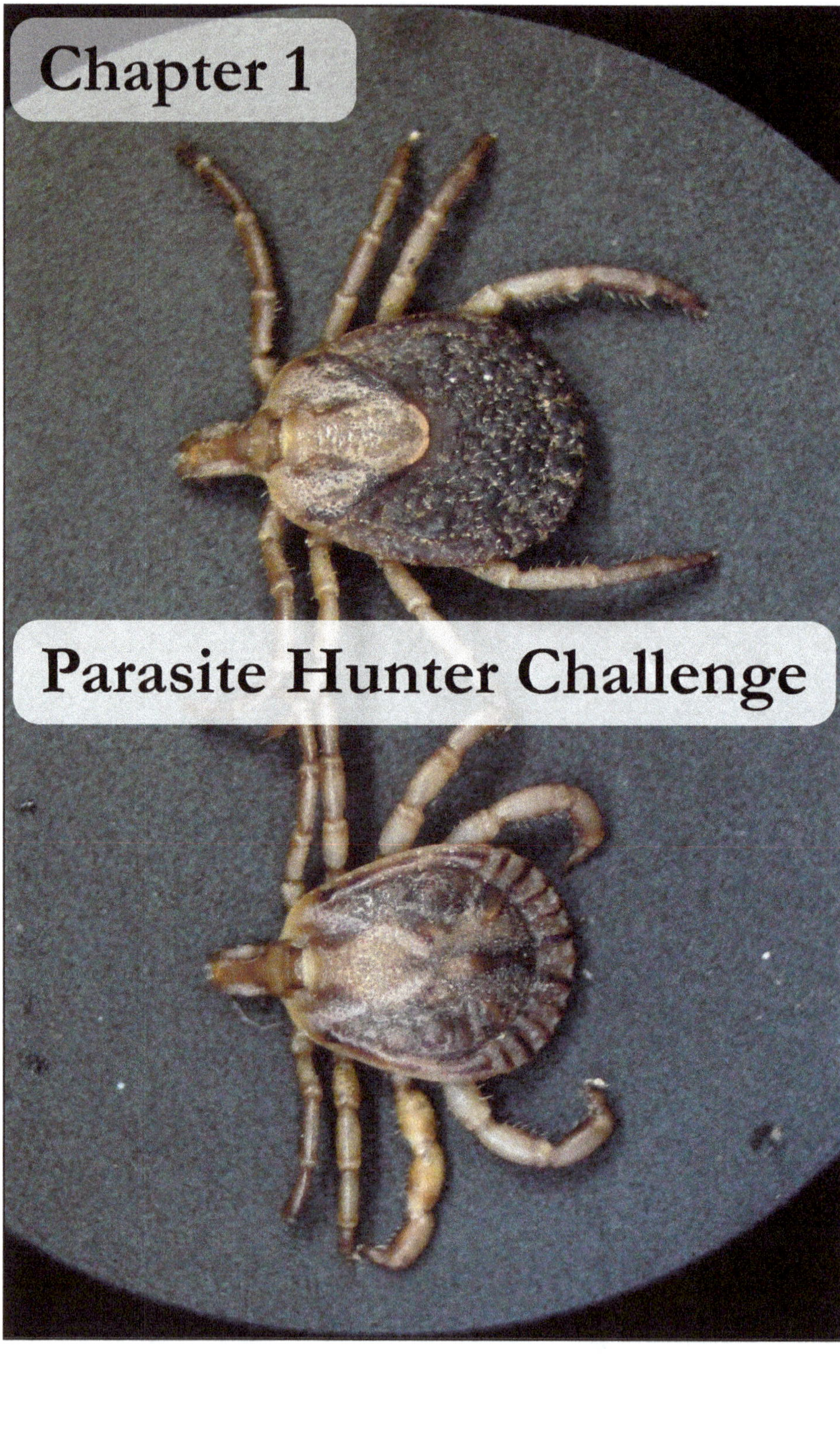

Join the Adventure - Author's Note – Your Journey Begins Here

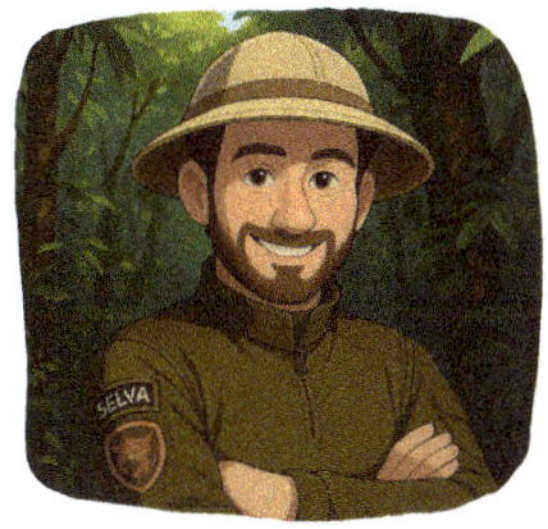

Welcome, brave explorer!

This is not just a book—it's a real adventure into the mysterious world of parasites!

To begin your journey, scan the QR Code on the next page (15) and watch the first video. In it, a mystery begins to unfold deep in the heart of the Amazon. But this is no ordinary story—you are a key part of it.

Your first mission?

Search through the pages of this book and find the hidden coordinates. These will lead you to a very special place—where, in the year 2000, a scientific expedition set out to hunt for ticks among the forest shadows.

Decipher this clue, and you will unlock the second step in your adventure.

The Parasite Hunter Challenge

This book contains 10 secret challenges—each one a puzzle, a clue, or a test of your observation skills.

What can you expect?

- QR codes linked to exclusive videos from the Amazon rainforest.
- "Where is the parasite?" photo challenges: Search detailed images and find the hidden parasite

- Pages that hold mysteries between the lines—from codes, coordinates, to animal tracks
- A final challenge that will reveal a hidden link… a direct portal to speak with the author himself!

Rewards for the Best Parasite Hunters

If you make it to the end and solve the mystery, you'll unlock:

✔ Access to a private VIP group with the author, Flávio Terassini

✔ A personal chat link to ask your questions and share your discoveries

✔ Downloadable exclusive photos of rare parasites from the Amazon

✔ The chance to become a real-life Parasite Hunter—recognized by Flávio himself

This is more than learning—it's discovery through curiosity, observation, and fun.

- So grab a pencil, scan those codes, search every image, and unlock a world that few have ever seen.
- Do you have what it takes to complete the hunt?
- Let the Parasite Hunter Challenge begin!

The Parasite Dice Game - Have fun and learn:

- Roll the dice and embark on a fun parasite-themed adventure—use a real die or a dice app on your phone!

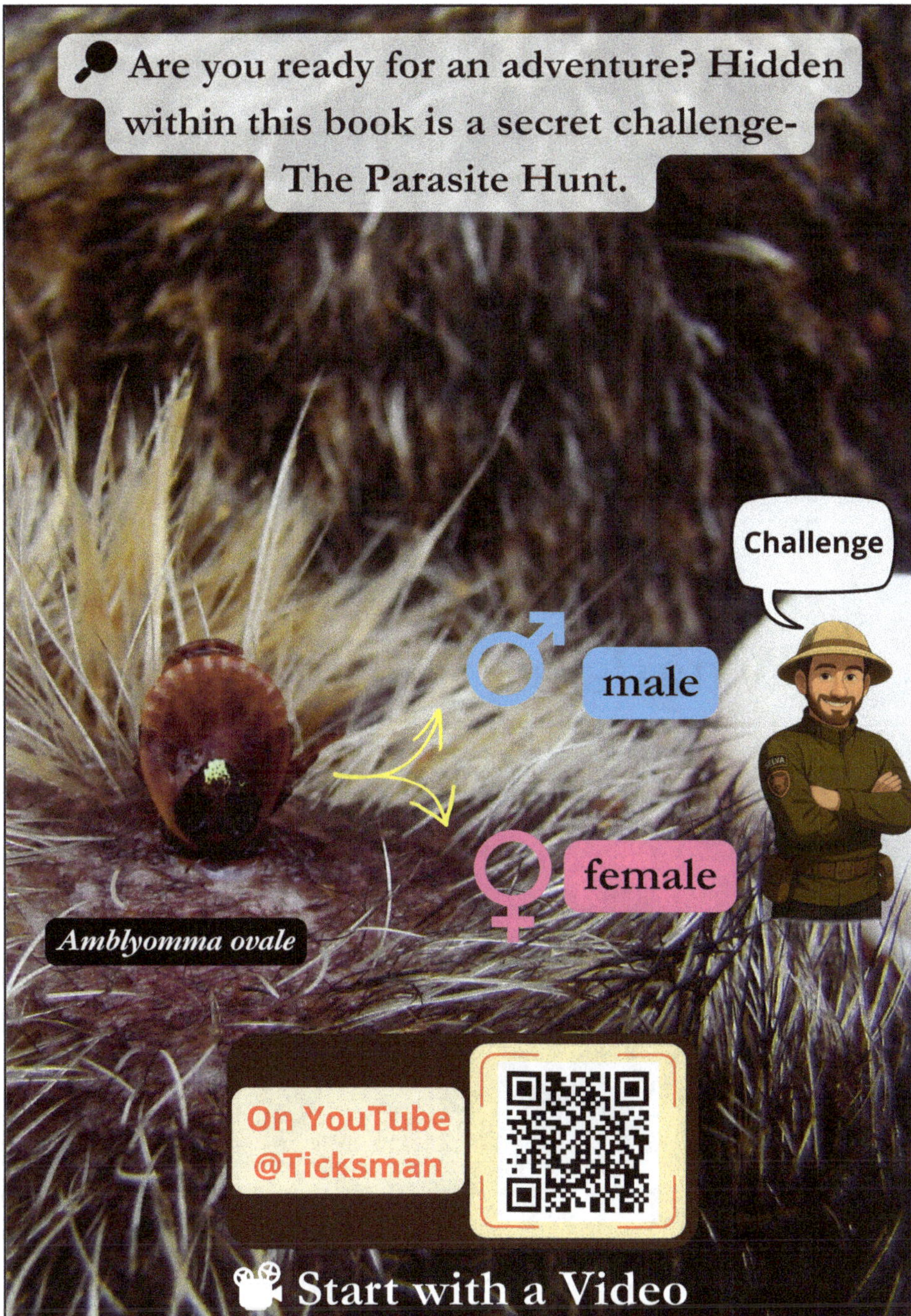
Are you ready for an adventure? Hidden within this book is a secret challenge- The Parasite Hunt.
Challenge
male
female
Amblyomma ovale
On YouTube
@Ticksman
Start with a Video

Spotted on the side of BR-364 near Ariquemes, Rondônia: a tick firmly attached to a carnivorous mammal after a roadkill incident. Ticks can detect body heat and carbon dioxide from far away—once they latch on, they feed for several days without letting go.

Chapter 2

What's so fascinating about Tropical Parasites?

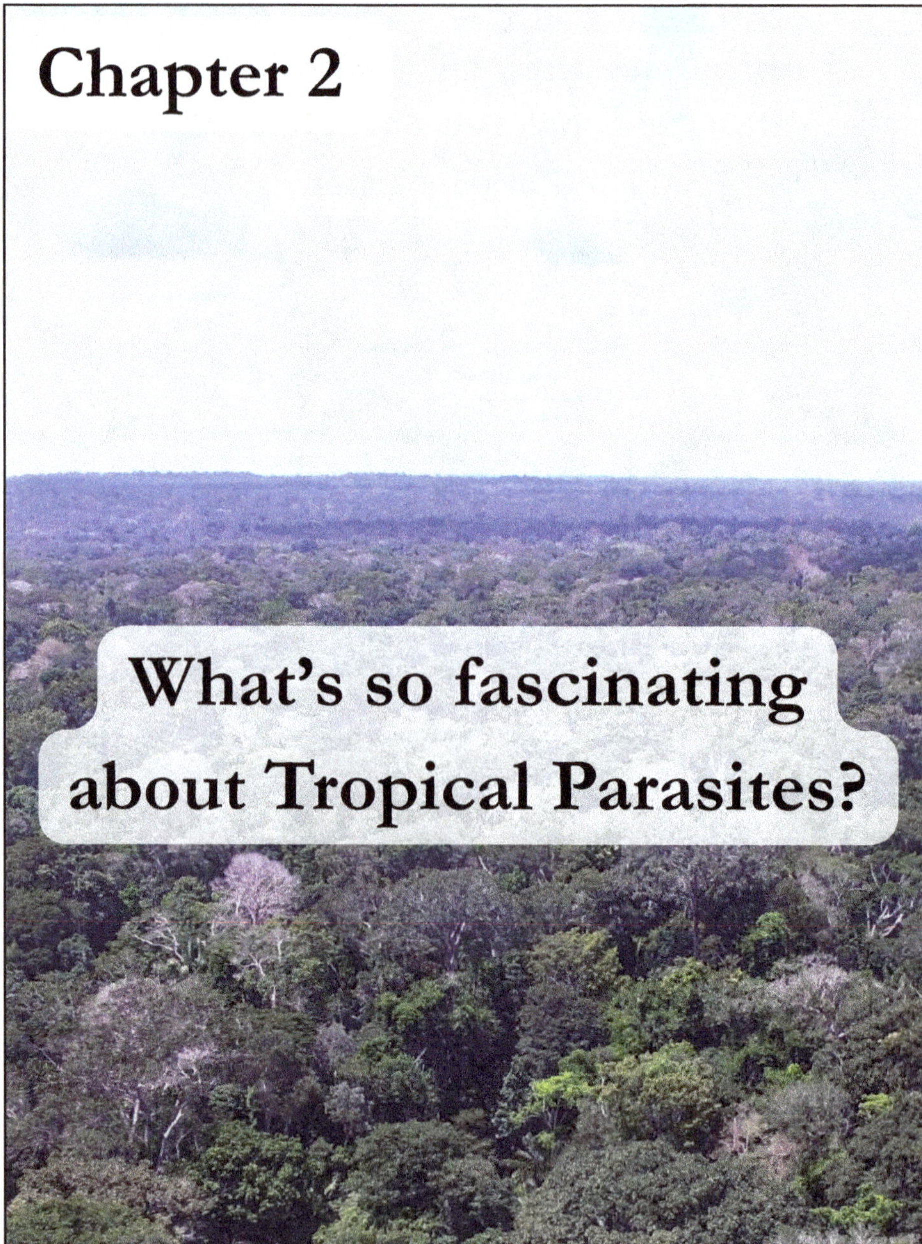

Aerial image captured by drone over the Samuel Ecological Station, located in Candeias do Jamari, Rondônia. This expansive forest canopy conceals an immense biodiversity—countless trees form complex ecological layers, each supporting a wide array of animal species. The sheer number of organisms thriving in this protected area highlights the critical role such ecosystems play in sustaining Amazonian biodiversity.

Parasites are organisms that survive at the expense of other living beings—sometimes causing harm, sometimes not. They take what they need—food, shelter, a place to live, and even a way to move around—without having to work for it or spend any energy.

This group includes both plants and animals and is divided into ectoparasites (external) and endoparasites (internal). Some of the most well-known parasites are ticks, lice, fleas, assassin bugs, bed bugs, and leeches. Others live inside their hosts, like roundworms, tapeworms, and schistosomes.

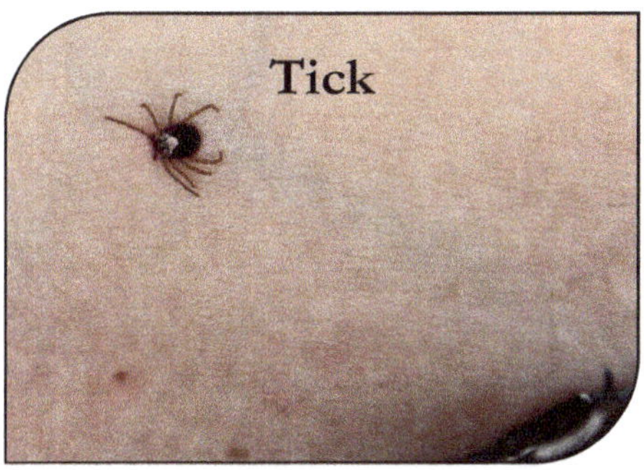

ectoparasites

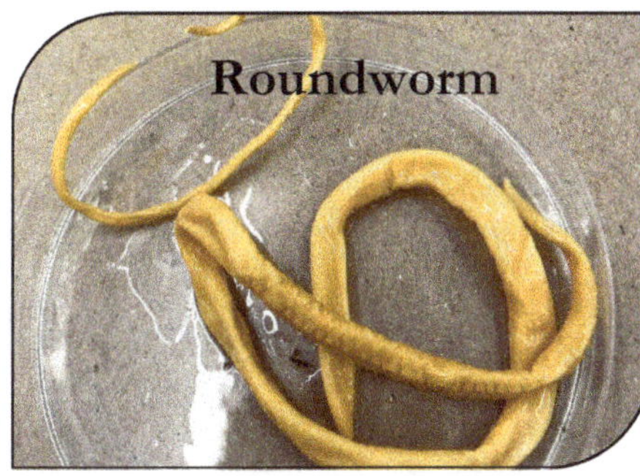

endoparasites

But parasites don't live alone! They rely on hosts—their living "homes"—to survive. Some even hitch a ride on vectors, nature's little "vehicles" that transport parasites from one place to another. And then there are the pathogens, the feared microbes responsible for some of the most notorious diseases on Earth.

In this book, we'll dive deep into the biology and ecology of these fascinating (and sometimes terrifying) creatures. We'll uncover their secrets—how they live, spread, and interact with the world around them. We'll explore their warning signs, symptoms, and modes of transmission, but most importantly, we'll focus on the one thing even more crucial than treatment: prevention.

After all, parasites have been around since the age of dinosaurs—and some species even predate them! They are masters of survival, highly specialized or cunningly adaptable, resilient, and, in some cases, nearly indestructible. But knowledge is power! By understanding how they work, we can learn to avoid, prevent, and even control them in our homes, workplaces, and daily lives.

So, are you ready for this journey into the microscopic (and sometimes not-so-microscopic) world of parasites? Let's dive in! But be careful not to be found.

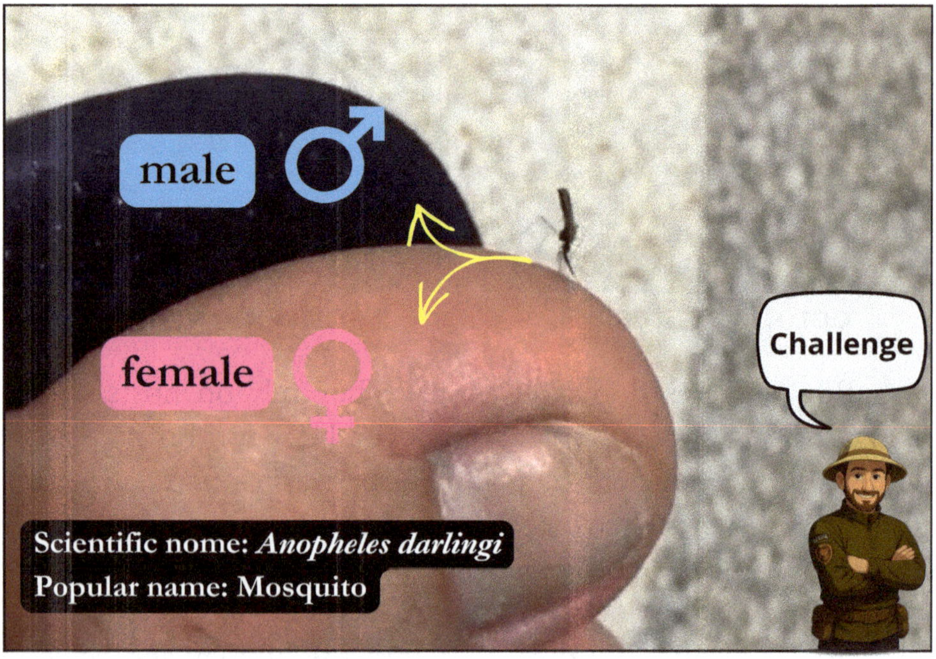
male ♂
female ♀
Challenge
Scientific nome: *Anopheles darlingi*
Popular name: Mosquito

A mosquito (*Anopheles darlingi*) feeding on the author's toe while he was having Sunday dinner at his parents' home in Porto Velho, Rondônia. These mosquitoes can detect a potential host from several meters away by sensing carbon dioxide and body heat. Once close, they search for an exposed area—like the leg, arm, or neck—where they can begin feeding on blood, a nutrient-rich meal. During this process, the mosquito injects saliva that contains anesthetics (so the bite isn't felt), anticoagulants, and vasodilators to ensure smooth feeding. However, if the mosquito is infected, this very saliva can transmit malaria and other diseases to the host.

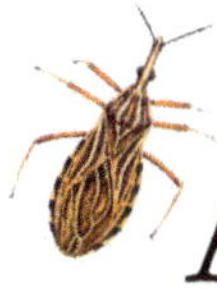

Tiny, Dangerous, and Absolutely Fascinating!

Parasites come in all shapes and sizes, but most of them are small—some, like mites, are microscopic, measuring just a few millimeters. Others, like ticks, are stealthy, silent, and capable of hiding just about anywhere.

They are dangerous because they transmit a wide range of diseases caused by bacteria, viruses, protozoa, and worms. In fact, over 4 billion people—half of the world's population—live in areas at risk of contracting a parasitic disease. And the numbers are alarming: every year, more than 2 million people die worldwide due to parasitic infections.

But parasites are also fascinating. They have been on this planet for hundreds of millions of years—long before the dinosaurs. They thrive in nearly every environment imaginable: savannas, rainforests, deserts, temperate regions, swamps, and beyond. Some live inside organisms, while others remain outside, clinging to their hosts. They are highly adaptable, resilient, and nearly indestructible.

Most parasites rely on their highly developed sensory organs to detect their hosts. And their favorite food? Blood! For many species, especially females, blood is the ultimate energy source, packed with nutrients that allow them to reproduce and lay eggs.

And while many parasites are tiny, some are gigantic—like the tapeworm (Taenia), which can grow up to 25 meters (82 feet) long inside a single human host!

They are mysterious, incredible, and sometimes terrifying. But one thing is certain: learning about them is not only fun—it's essential!

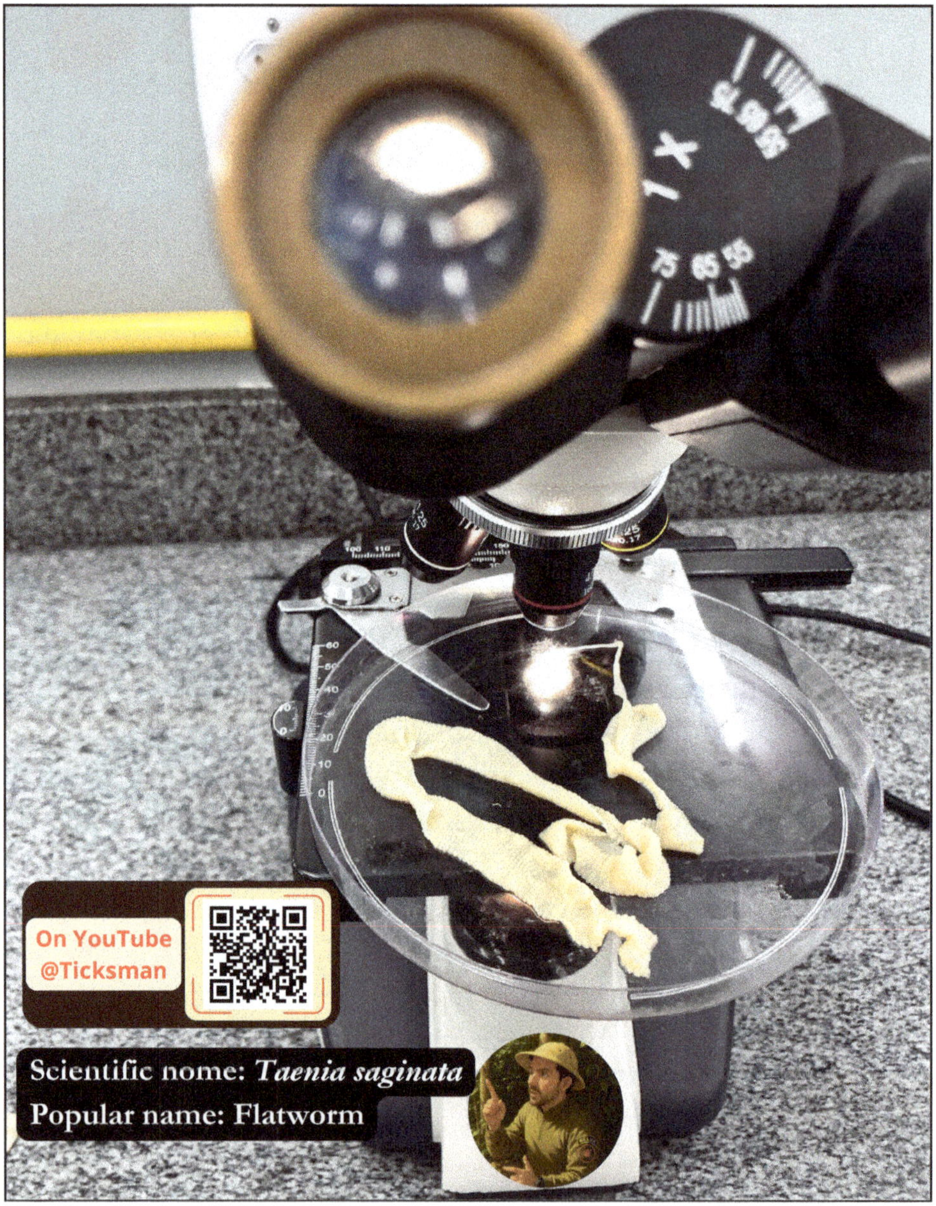
On YouTube
@Ticksman
Scientific nome: *Taenia saginata*
Popular name: Flatworm

Taenia saginata, a beef tapeworm, being prepared for microscopic observation in the lab. This specimen was surprisingly found in the diaper of a 2-year-old child in Porto Velho, Rondônia—and gifted to the author by a friend working at a local hospital. Parasites can show up in the most unexpected places. Tapeworms are often sneaky and, in many cases, asymptomatic—meaning you could be reading this book while being infected without even knowing it. That's why it's so important to visit a doctor regularly and perform routine health check-ups, including blood, urine, and of course, stool exams.

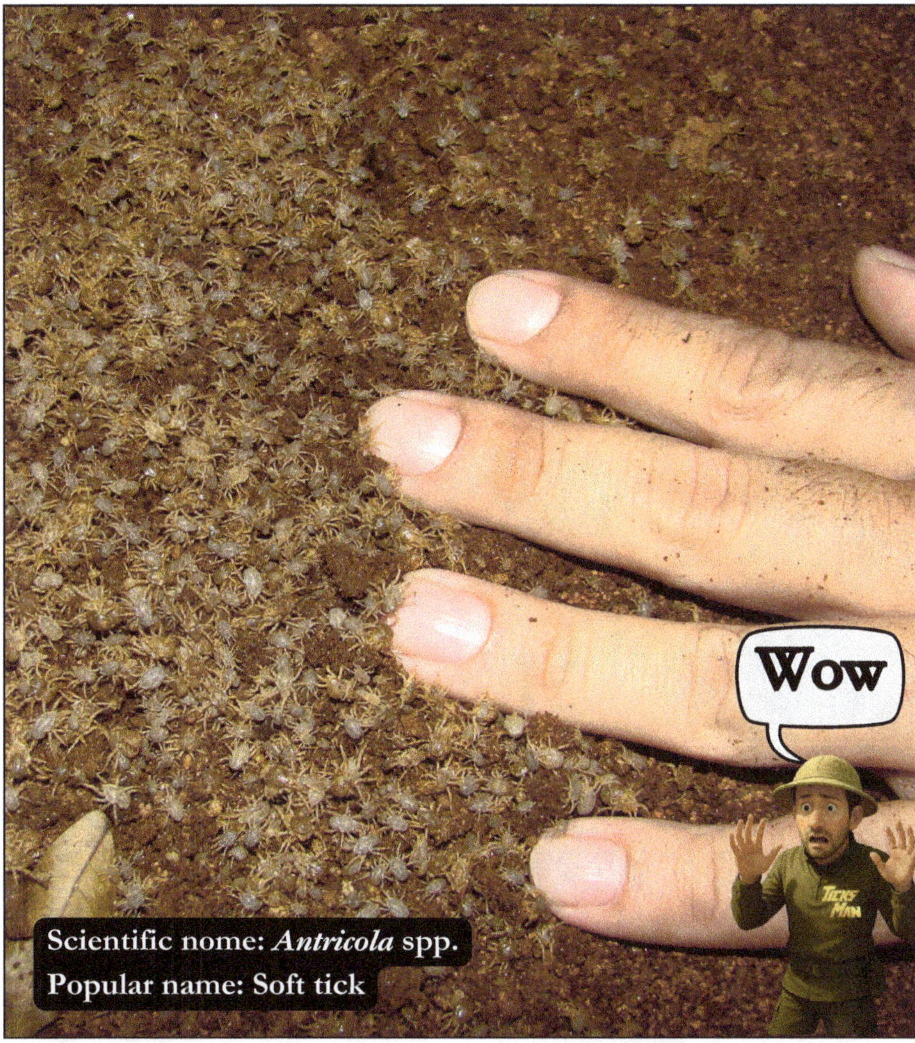

On YouTube @Ticksman

On TikTok @Ticksman

One of the highest known concentrations of ticks in the Amazon Rainforest—millions of Argasidae family ticks discovered deep inside a cave. Scientific expeditions have been carried out here since 2002, and you can watch two special videos documenting the author's research in this exact location. Get ready to explore the cave where the ticks rule.

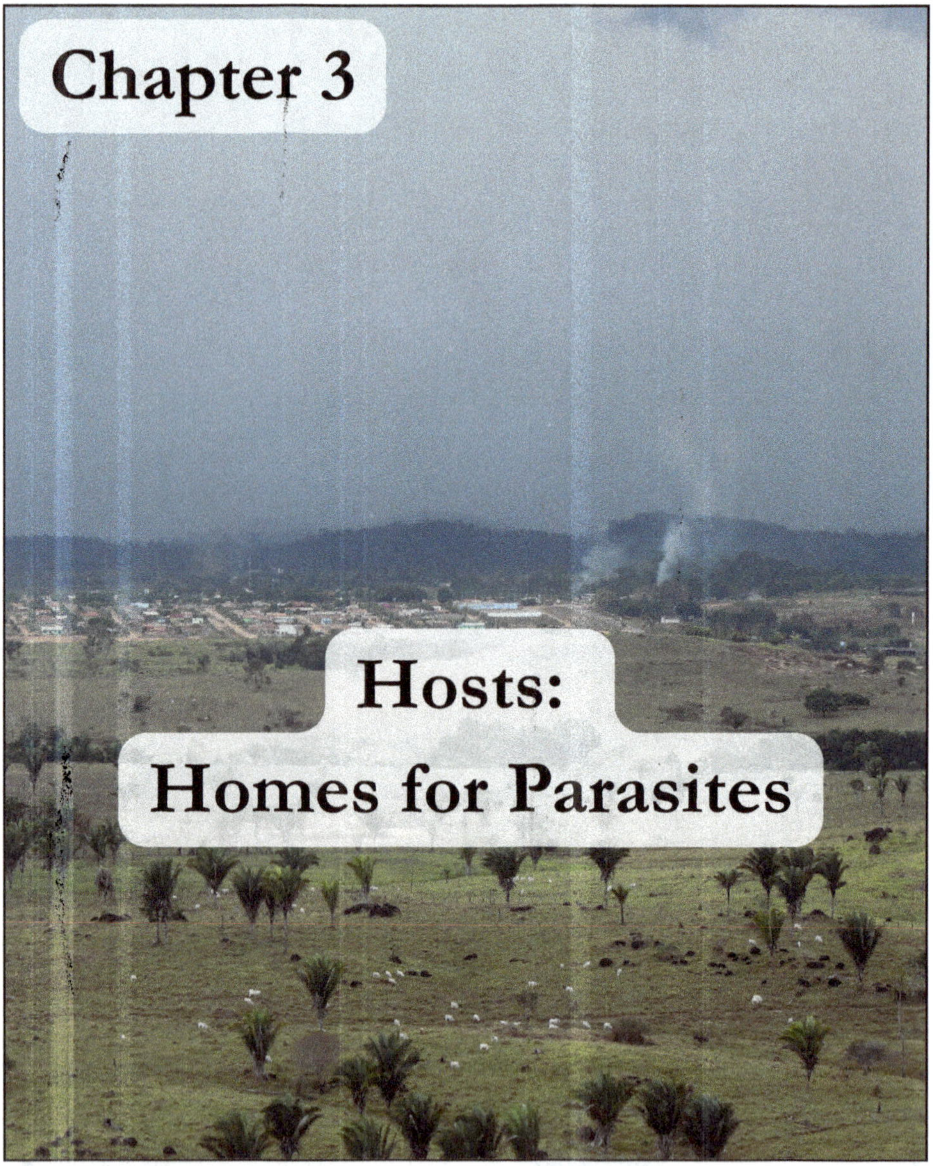

Although a rural town, Monte Negro, can be seen in the distance—about 250 km (approximately 155 miles) from Porto Velho, the capital of Rondônia—notice the abundance of babassu palms, a common and resilient tree species thriving in pastures across the region. In studies on Chagas disease transmission, researchers found an average of 20 insect vectors per babassu tree. This town holds special meaning for the author, who lived here for five years and began his journey in tropical disease research in 1999 as a research intern at the University of São Paulo's Institute of Biomedical Sciences (ICB5).

To better understand how parasites interact with their hosts and transmit diseases, we will use ticks as a model.

Ticks feed on the blood of a horse that is contaminated with a pathogen, and by biting another host, they transmit the disease. This simple yet deadly process illustrates the intricate relationship between hosts, vectors, and pathogens—a key concept we'll explore throughout this book.

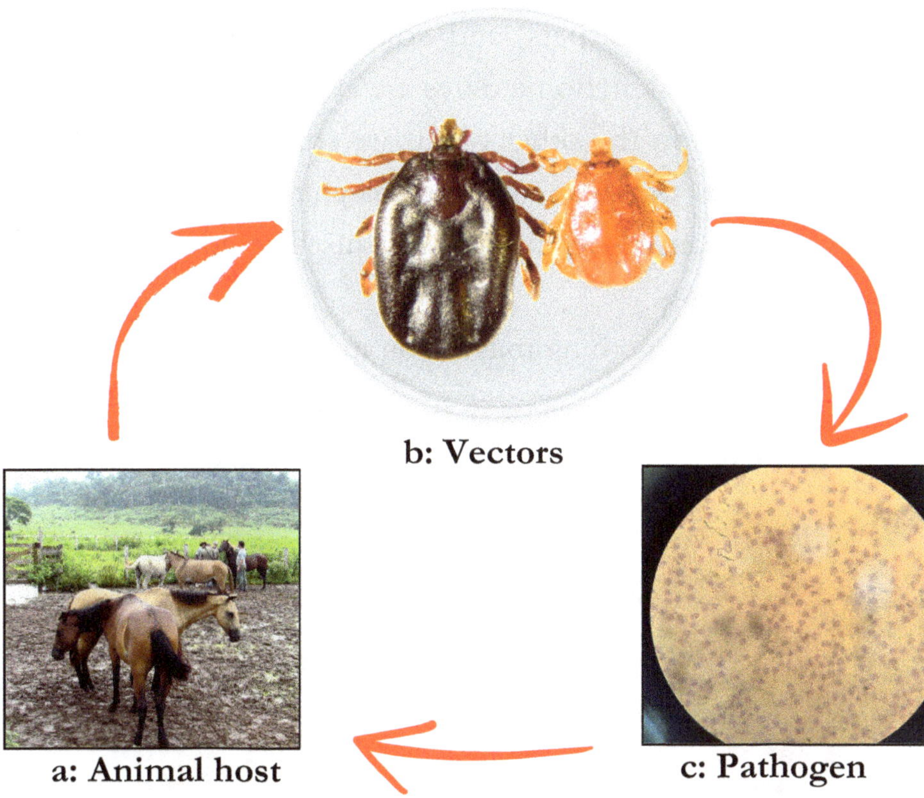

In the parasite transmission cycle, vectors (like ticks), animal hosts (such as horses), and pathogens (such as *Babesia* spp.) each play a vital role in the spread of disease. When a tick like *Dermacentor nitens* feeds on a host—often attaching to a horse's ears—it can become infected with a pathogen. This pathogen may not always be Babesia; it could also be a bacterium, virus, or another parasite. A few days later, when the tick bites another animal—or even a human—it may transmit the infection. The new host can become positive for the disease, sometimes showing symptoms within a short period, or sometimes remaining asymptomatic for a long time.

For example - Tiny But Not the Same: Mites vs. Tick Larvae

Many people call both mites and tick larvae by the same name: "micuim". But they are actually very different!

Mites are super tiny—you can't see them with your eyes. They live in grass, carpets, and sofas, and they often cause allergies and itchy skin. Some mites are even microscopic!

Tick larvae, on the other hand, are small but visible. They have three pairs of legs, and after hatching, they crawl onto animals or humans to feed on blood. Just like adult ticks, they can spread diseases.

So next time something makes you itchy—remember, not all "micuins" are the same!

Mite

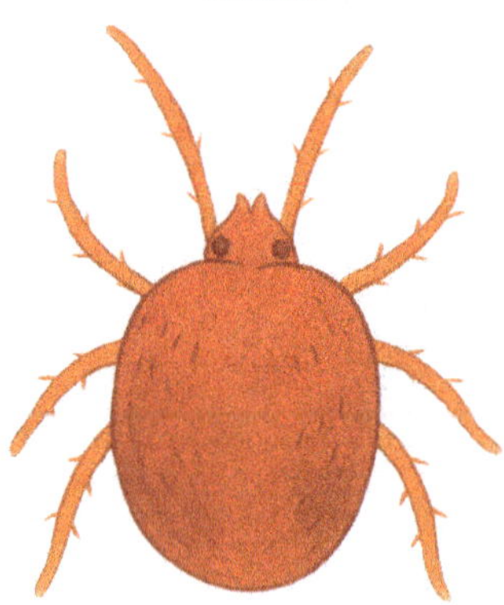

Tick

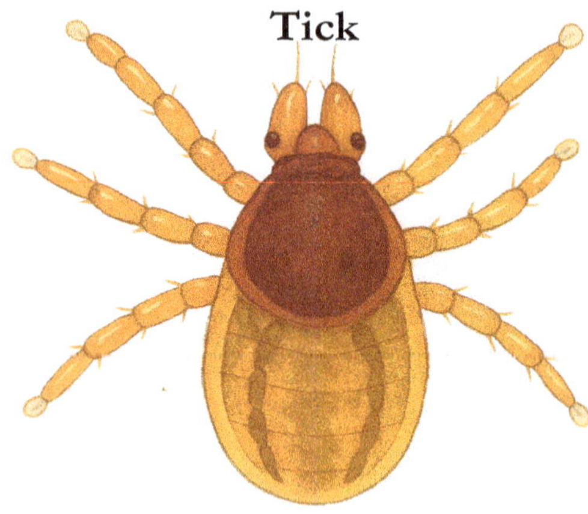

Take a closer look! On the left, you'll see an adult Trombiculidae mite with four legs on each side—tiny and almost invisible to the naked eye. Beside it is a tick larva, slightly larger, with only three legs on each side. Although they both belong to the mighty mite family, only the tick larva feeds on blood! While the Trombiculidae mite mainly causes skin irritation and allergies, the tick larva can become a true traveler, jumping to animals or humans in search of a blood meal. It's amazing how such tiny creatures can have such different lifestyles!

Wild Hosts X Domestic Hosts

Hosts are those animals (preferably vertebrates) that harbor or carry the pathogens. They may be asymptomatic and not show any signs or symptoms of contamination. However, it is not advantageous for the pathogen to kill its host, as it may also die. See how many we can contact.

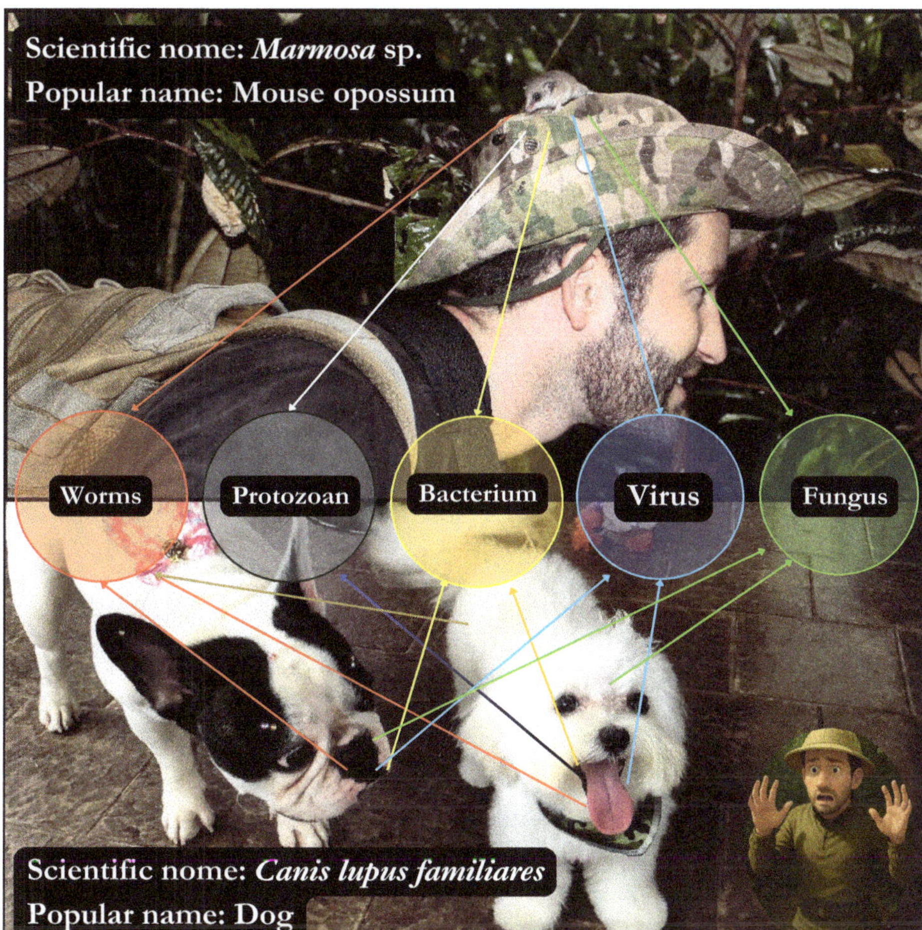
Scientific nome: *Marmosa* sp.
Popular name: Mouse opossum
Worms
Protozoan
Bacterium
Virus
Fungus
Scientific nome: *Canis lupus familiares*
Popular name: Dog

A true Amazon moment—while deep in the rainforest, a curious marsupial dropped right onto the author's hat! Below, meet his loyal companions: Amora and Pudim, the family's beloved pets. "*Uta Ixicum Coteca Trama Catim.*"

Wild Hosts: Nature's Reservoirs

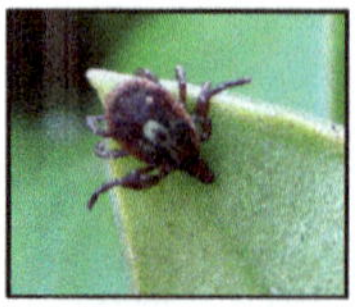

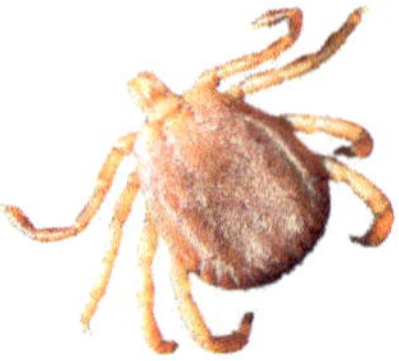

Parasites need a home, and for many of them, that home is a host—a living organism that shelters and nourishes both external and internal parasites. Some of these hosts live in savannas, forests, jungles, swamps, and deserts, while others have adapted to urban environments, becoming synanthropic animals—wild creatures that coexist with humans, often turning into pests. Rodents, opossums, and bats are prime examples of animals that thrive in cities, bringing parasites with them.

Many wild animals, also known as reservoir hosts, help maintain parasite populations in nature. Species like peccaries (South American wild boars) and armadillos, for instance, can become infected by parasites, bacteria, viruses, fungi, and protozoa in several ways:

- Foraging on the ground, where they ingest contaminated food or decomposing organic matter.
- Drinking water from natural reservoirs polluted with feces and urine from infected animals.
- Being bitten or stung by insects and arachnids that carry pathogens in their saliva or feces.

Once inside a new host, the biological cycle continues. The microorganisms feed, reproduce, and multiply, making this new body their home. Over time, many wild animals develop immune resistance, allowing them to coexist with these parasites without falling ill. However, some are not as fortunate and succumb to infections.

These reservoir hosts play a crucial role in sustaining the life cycle of various pathogens in the wild. Under natural conditions, without human interference, this cycle remains balanced. But when deforestation, fires, habitat destruction, and other human-induced environmental changes occur, equilibrium is lost. This disruption often leads to disease outbreaks, ranging from:

- **Endemics**, where infections persist in localized areas.
- **Epidemics**, affecting larger regions such as states, provinces, or neighboring countries.
- **Pandemics**, where outbreaks spread across continents, impacting populations worldwide.

Nature has its way of keeping things in balance, but when we interfere, the consequences can be devastating. Understanding the role of wild hosts in parasitic cycles is key to preventing future health crises.

And so we have a big problem. Diseases.

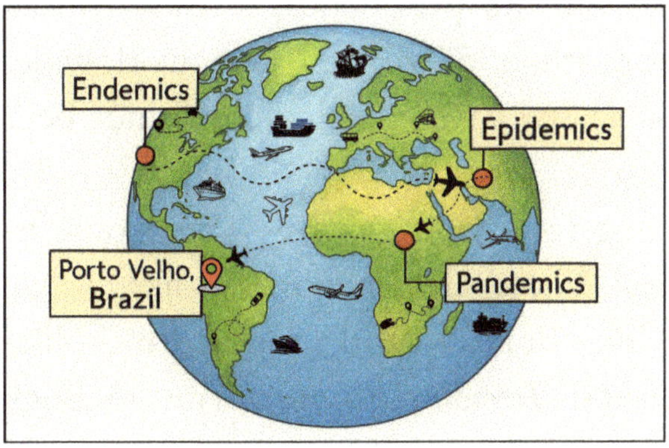

Biopiracy:
With the growing global interest in exotic species, many animals and plants are being introduced into new environments—sometimes illegally. As a result, new diseases are emerging in places where they previously did not exist. So, stay alert and be responsible. Prevention starts with awareness.

This map illustrates the difference between endemic, epidemic, and pandemic disease patterns. An endemic remains restricted to a specific area; an epidemic spreads across larger regions; and a pandemic crosses international borders, affecting multiple continents. After witnessing recent global events, it's worth asking: How can we prevent the next pandemic? The answer begins with science, education, vigilance, and global cooperation.

Diseases Carried by Wild Animals

This table presents five major parasitic diseases for each of the main pathogen groups: **worms, protozoa, bacteria, viruses**, and **fungi**. It includes their common names, scientific names, and the animals that act as hosts, reservoirs, or carriers —those that help spread the infection.

I. **Worms (Helminths)**

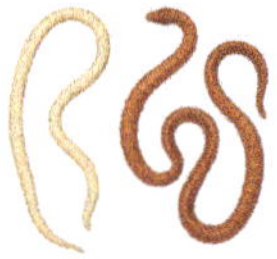

The most widespread worms in the world are transmitted via the "fecal-oral" route—meaning human feces contaminate water or food. One prime example is the roundworm Ascaris lumbricoides. Some studies suggest that 4 out of every 10 people have had, or currently have, this worm. In fact, about 50% of the global population—over 4 billion people—live in areas at risk. However, despite its prevalence, Ascaris causes relatively few deaths: fewer than 5,000 per year worldwide. Since this worm is not associated with a vector, it will not be a focus in our book.

Now here's a fascinating fact about worms: They come in many shapes and lifestyles! There are flatworms—like *Taenia* (tapeworms) and *Fasciola* (liver flukes)—and roundworms—like *Ancylostoma* (hookworms) and *Toxocara* (roundworms in dogs and cats). Some are internal parasites (endoparasites), while others live freely in soil or water, like the simple yet amazing planarians. Fossils show that worms have existed long before the age of dinosaurs, and they have adapted to every imaginable habitat.

Here's something to think about: Scientists estimate there could be over 24 million different species of living organisms on Earth. If each one hosts even a single unique type of parasitic worm… we could be looking at 24 million different worm species! That would make worms the most diverse group of living beings on the planet. Eureka!

I've selected what I consider to be the five most important parasitic diseases—each one linked to zoonotic transmission or arthropod vectors, whether through saliva, feces, or mechanical transfer via their legs, antennae, or body surface. One of these diseases will be explored in greater detail based on its relevance, symptoms, severity, or its potential to spread to humans.

This table presents: the Common Name of the Disease, the Scientific Name of the Pathogen, and the Animals that Carry or Host the Parasite.

Common Name of the Disease	Scientific Name	Animals that Carry or Host the Parasite
*Hydatid Disease (Echinococcosis)	*Echinococcus granulosus / E. multilocularis*	Wild canids: wolves, foxes
Trichinellosis	*Trichinella spiralis / T. nativa*	Wild boars, bears, walruses
Raccoon Roundworm Infection	*Baylisascaris procyonis*	Raccoons
Giant Kidney Worm Infection	*Dioctophyme renale*	Mink, otters, wild canids
Rat Lungworm Disease	*Angiostrongylus cantonensis*	Rats (host), snails and slugs (vector)

*See example on next page

*Hydatid Disease (Echinococcosis)

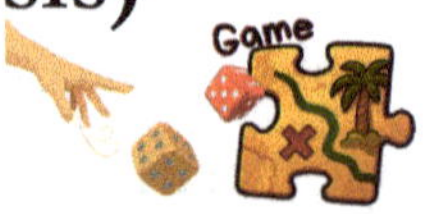

Transmission / Vectors

The disease is spread when people accidentally swallow tiny parasite eggs. These eggs come from the poop of infected dogs or wild canids like foxes and wolves that ate infected organs of animals like sheep.

Signs and Symptoms

At first, there are usually no symptoms. But over time, big cysts (fluid-filled sacs) can grow inside organs like the liver or lungs, causing pain, coughing, or belly problems.

Diagnosis / Tests

Doctors use blood tests and imaging tools like ultrasound, CT scans, or X-rays to look for the cysts inside the body.

Prevention / Prophylaxis

Wash your hands after touching dogs or soil, don't let dogs eat raw organs from other animals, and deworm pets regularly.

Treatment

Some cases are treated with special medicine, but bigger cysts might need surgery to remove them safely. A doctor will confirm the diagnosis and begin the correct treatment. Do not self-medicate.

Geographic Distribution

This disease is more common in rural or farming areas in South America, Eastern Europe, Africa, and Central Asia—especially where people live close to dogs and livestock.

Worms That Threaten Us: A Global Overview

The table below highlights four important helminthic diseases linked to wild animals. These infections, though rare in some regions, can cause serious harm to humans if not properly diagnosed and treated. By learning about their transmission, symptoms, and prevention, we can better protect ourselves—especially when traveling or exploring nature.

Characteristics	Trichinellosis	Raccoon Roundworm Infection	Giant Kidney Worm Infection	Rat Lungworm Disease
Transmission / Vectors	Undercooked pork or wild game	Ingestion of contaminated soil or feces (from raccoons)	Ingestion of raw/ undercooked fish or frogs	Ingestion of snails/slugs or contaminated vegetables
Signs and Symptoms	Muscle pain, fever, swelling, diarrhea	Nerve damage, blindness, coma	Kidney damage, abdominal pain	Headache, stiff neck, nausea, neurological symptoms
Diagnosis / Tests	Blood test, muscle biopsy	Clinical signs, serology	Urine test, imaging	CSF analysis, PCR, serology
Prevention / Prophylaxis	Cook meat thoroughly	Avoid soil contact, wash hands	Avoid raw freshwater animals	Wash produce, avoid raw snails/slugs
Treatment	Seek medical help; treatment exists	Seek medical help; supportive care	Seek medical help; surgery may be needed	Seek medical help; treatment exists
Geographic Distribution	Cosmopolitan (especially in rural areas)	North America	North America, Europe, Asia	Southeast Asia, Pacific Islands, Americas

Protozoan diseases can be transmitted to humans in many ways: through contaminated water, food, insect vectors, from mother to child (transplacental), accidental exposure in laboratories, blood transfusions, and organ transplants from infected donors. Some species may also enter through mucous membranes or breaks in the skin.

These microorganisms are clever, highly adaptable, and capable of surviving in diverse climates and extreme environments. Long before the dinosaurs walked the Earth, protozoa were already here—making them one of the oldest forms of life on the planet. Controlling them remains one of science's greatest challenges.

Let's dive deeper into the fascinating world of protozoa.

II. Protozoan Diseases

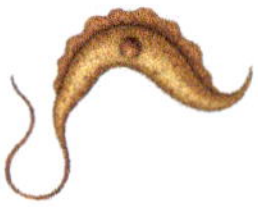

Common Name of the Disease	Scientific Name	Animals that Carry or Host the Parasite
*Malaria	*Plasmodium* spp.	Monkeys (in some regions)
*Chagas Disease	*Trypanosoma cruzi*	Opossums, armadillos, rodents
Leishmaniasis	*Leishmania* spp.	Rodents, wild canids, marsupials
Toxoplasmosis	*Toxoplasma gondii*	Wild felines, rodents
Babesiosis	*Babesia* spp.	Deer and rodents (transmitted by ticks)

*See example following pages

*Malaria Disease (*Plasmodium* spp.)

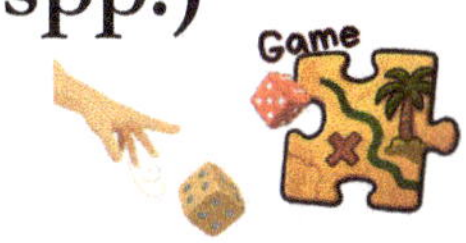

Transmission / Vectors

Malaria is spread by the bite of a female mosquito called *Anopheles*. She carries the parasite in her saliva and passes it on when she drinks blood.

Signs and Symptoms

The person may feel very tired, have high fever, chills, headaches, and sometimes vomit. The symptoms can come in waves.

Diagnosis / Tests

Doctors look at a drop of blood under the microscope to find the parasite. There are also quick tests that work like a COVID test.

Prevention / Prophylaxis

Use mosquito nets, wear long clothes, and put on repellent. In some places, people take special pills before visiting areas with malaria.

Treatment

Malaria is treated with medicines that kill the parasite in the blood. The treatment must be started quickly to avoid serious problems. A doctor will confirm the diagnosis and begin the correct treatment. Do not self-medicate.

Geographic Distribution

Malaria is found mostly in tropical areas like parts of Africa, Asia, and the Amazon region in South America.

Chagas Disease (*Trypanosoma cruzi*)

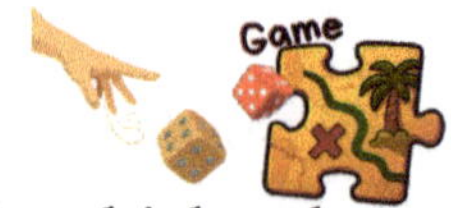

Transmission / Vectors

Transmitted by assassin bugs (Triatomines), which release infected feces while feeding on blood. The parasite enters through the bite site or mucous membranes. Can also spread via blood transfusion, organ transplants, from mother to baby, or through contaminated food or lab accidents.

Signs and Symptoms

In the acute phase: fever, fatigue, body aches, and swelling near the bite (Romaña's sign near the eye). In the chronic phase (which may last for decades): heart or digestive system complications—sometimes fatal.

Diagnosis / Tests

Blood tests (microscopy, ELISA, PCR) are used to detect the parasite. Chronic cases require serological testing.

Prevention / Prophylaxis

Avoid sleeping in mud, adobe, or thatched houses in endemic areas. Keep homes sealed and clean. Screen windows and use insecticides. Ensure safe food handling. Blood donors should be screened.

Treatment

Treatment exists and is most effective in the early stages. Always consult a doctor immediately if exposed or symptomatic. Chronic cases require long-term monitoring.

Geographic Distribution

Endemic in rural parts of Latin America. Increasing cases in the U.S., Europe, and Asia due to migration—often undiagnosed in non-endemic regions.

Microscopic but Mighty: Protozoan Parasites that Affect Millions

This table highlights four of the most important protozoan diseases affecting humans. These tiny single-celled organisms can cause silent infections—or severe illness, depending on the host's health and the pathogen's aggressiveness. Whether transmitted by insects, food, or congenital means, protozoans are a major concern in both rural and urban settings. Learning how they spread and how to protect ourselves is the first step in defeating them.

Characteristics	Leishmaniasis	Toxoplasmosis	Babesiosis
Transmission / Vectors	Bite of infected sandflies; dog reservoirs	Ingestion of oocysts (cat feces, raw meat); congenital	Bite of infected ticks (e.g., Ixodidae)
Signs and Symptoms	Skin ulcers, fever, enlarged organs (visceral form)	Often asymptomatic; fever, headache, risk for fetus and immunocompromised	Fever, chills, fatigue, anemia
Diagnosis / Tests	Blood test, tissue biopsy, PCR	Serology, PCR, prenatal screening	Blood smear, PCR, serology
Prevention / Prophylaxis	Insecticide-treated nets, avoid outdoor exposure in endemic areas	Avoid raw meat, wash produce, clean litter boxes with gloves	Tick control, avoid tick habitats
Treatment	Exists for all forms; must be guided by a doctor	Depends on severity and immune status; see a doctor	Antiprotozoal treatment under supervision
Geographic Distribution	Tropical/subtropical regions worldwide	Worldwide; high in areas with cats and raw meat consumption	U.S., Europe, parts of Asia and Africa

Just like protozoa, bacteria are incredibly adaptable and can thrive in nearly every environment on Earth—from freezing cold regions to extreme heat. Some bacteria have even been found in volcanic lava, such as Thermus aquaticus, which survives in boiling hot springs. Whether in mountain peaks or ocean depths, inside or outside plants and animals—bacteria are everywhere. To give you an idea, nearly 2 kilograms (about 4.4 pounds) of the average human body weight is made up of bacteria. These microorganisms live in harmony with us and play essential roles, such as helping with digestion.

However, there's a serious warning: NEVER self-medicate with antibiotics without consulting a doctor. When antibiotics are misused or overused, bacteria "learn" to survive and adapt.

Only the strongest, most resistant ones remain, leading to the rise of dangerous superbugs. In this chapter, we'll explore some of the bacteria that are transmitted by animals and vectors—tiny creatures with the power to cause big problems. Let's find out more about them!

III. Bacterial Diseases

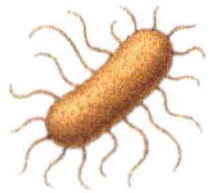

Common Name of the Disease	Scientific Name	Animals that Carry or Host the Parasite
*Plague	*Yersinia pestis*	Rodents (transmitted by fleas)
Lyme Disease	*Borrelia burgdorferi*	Deer, rodents (transmitted by ticks)
Rocky Mountain Spotted Fever (RMSF)	*Rickettsia rickettsii*	Wild mammals (transmitted by ticks)
Leptospirosis	*Leptospira* spp.	Rodents (by urine)
Brucellosis	*Brucella suis / B. melitensis*	Wild boars, bison, deer

*See example on next page

*Plague Disease (*Yersinia pestis*)

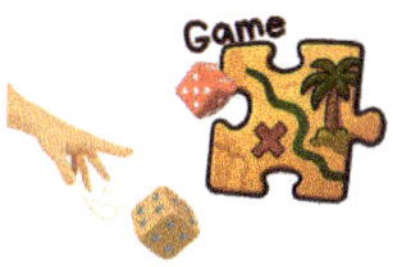

Transcription / Vectors

Plague is mostly spread by fleas that bite infected rodents (like rats) and then bite humans. It can also spread through contact with infected animals or, in rare cases, through the air from a person with lung infection.

Signs and Symptoms

There are different types of plague! The most common is bubonic plague, which causes fever, chills, weakness, and swollen painful lymph nodes (called "buboes"). Other types affect the lungs or blood.

Diagnosis / Tests

Doctors can test blood, lymph fluid, or sputum (from the lungs) to look for the bacteria Yersinia pestis that causes plague.

Prevention / Prophylaxis

Avoid contact with wild rodents and don't touch dead animals. Keep your home clean and rodent-free. In some high-risk areas, flea control on pets is very important.

Treatment

Plague can be deadly if not treated quickly, but it can be cured with antibiotics when diagnosed early. A doctor will confirm the diagnosis and begin the correct treatment. Do not self-medicate.

Geographic Distribution

Plague still exists today in parts of Africa, Asia, and even the western United States. It's rare but can spread fast if not controlled.

Bacterial Zoonoses: Hidden Threats from Nature

This table presents four significant bacterial diseases transmitted by animals or arthropod vectors. Whether through tick bites, contaminated water, or direct contact with infected animals, these pathogens can cause serious illness in humans. Understanding how these diseases spread and how to prevent them is key to avoiding infections—especially in areas where humans and animals share close environments.

Characteristics	Lyme Disease	Rocky Mountain Spotted Fever (RMSF)	Leptospirosis	Brucellosis
Transmission / Vectors	Tick bite (*Ixodes* spp.)	Tick bite (*Amblyomma*, *Dermacentor* spp.)	Contact with urine from infected animals (dogs, pigs, cattle)	Contact with infected animal fluids, raw dairy, undercooked meat
Signs and Symptoms	Fever, fatigue, joint pain, skin rash (bull's-eye)	Fever, rash, muscle pain, vomiting	Fever, chills, muscle pain, kidney/liver damage	Fever, fatigue, joint pain, reproductive issues
Diagnosis / Tests	Blood test (ELISA, Western Blot)	Blood test, PCR	Blood or urine test, ELISA	Blood culture, serology (ELISA)
Prevention / Prophylaxis	Use tick repellents, wear long clothes, check for ticks	Avoid tick-infested areas, use repellents	Avoid contact with contaminated water, wear boots/gloves	Avoid raw dairy, wear PPE when handling animals
Treatment	Seek medical care; treatment available	Seek immediate medical attention; treatment exists	Medical evaluation needed; treatable	See a doctor; long-term treatment may be needed
Geographic Distribution	North America, Europe, Asia	Americas (esp. USA, Brazil)	Worldwide (esp. tropical/ subtropical areas)	Global, esp. in livestock regions (Mediterranean, Latin America, Asia)

IV. Viral Diseases

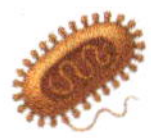

Viruses—these mysterious entities often seem like they came from outer space! In fact, some scientists have even called them "extraterrestrial-like" due to their bizarre structure and behavior. But what exactly are they? Viruses are complex and extremely clever. Once inside a host organism, they behave like classic parasites—hijacking the host's cellular machinery to replicate their own genetic material, whether it's DNA or RNA (yes, there are both DNA and RNA viruses!).

Sometimes, viruses go unnoticed, causing no symptoms at all. But other times, they are the culprits behind major global health crises. Just think of the last five major pandemics: COVID-19, H1N1 influenza (swine flu), SARS, MERS, and the ongoing seasonal flu outbreaks. In this book, however, we'll focus on the viruses that are transmitted by vectors or animals —those that jump from wildlife or domestic animals to humans, often with serious consequences. Let's explore these microscopic invaders and learn how to stay protected!

Common Name of the Disease	**Scientific Name**	**Animals that Carry or Host the Virus**
*Rabies	*Rabies virus*	Bats, foxes, raccoons, skunks, and other mammals
Hantavirus Pulmonary Syndrome (HPS)	*Hantavirus*	Rodents
Ebola Virus Disease	*Ebolavirus* spp.	Bats, primates
SARS (Severe Acute Respiratory Syndrome)	SARS-CoV	Bats, civet cats
MERS (Middle East Respiratory Syndrome)	MERS-CoV	Camels

*See example following pages

*Rabies Disease

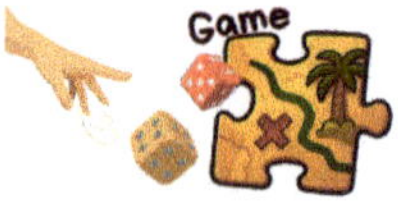

Transmission / Vectors

Rabies spreads through the saliva of infected animals—usually through a bite or scratch. Common carriers include dogs, bats, foxes, raccoons, and skunks.

Signs and Symptoms

Early signs include fever, tiredness, and pain near the bite. As it worsens, the person may have confusion, fear of water, trouble swallowing, and eventually lose control of muscles. Rabies always affects the brain.

Diagnosis / Tests

Rabies is very hard to confirm while a person is alive. Doctors use tests on saliva, skin, or spinal fluid—but mostly rely on history of animal bites and symptoms.

Prevention / Prophylaxis

Vaccination is the key! Pets and people who work with animals should be vaccinated. After a bite, quick treatment (post-exposure vaccine) can stop the virus before it reaches the brain.

Treatment

Once symptoms start, rabies is almost always fatal. That's why getting immediate medical help after a bite is so important. There is no cure once the disease begins.

Geographic Distribution

Rabies is found on every continent except Antarctica. It causes thousands of human deaths every year, especially in Asia and Africa, mostly from dog bites.

Viral Threats from Animals to Humans

This table highlights four of the most impactful viral diseases with zoonotic origins. Each is linked to animals—whether rodents, bats, camels, or primates—and can cause severe illness or global outbreaks. Understanding how they spread, how they affect the body, and where they are most commonly found is crucial for prevention. These viruses serve as a powerful reminder that public health and environmental awareness must go hand in hand.

Characteristics	Hantavirus Pulmonary Syndrome (HPS)	Ebola Virus Disease	SARS (Severe Acute Respiratory Syndrome)	MERS (Middle East Respiratory Syndrome)
Transmission / Vectors	Inhalation of rodent urine/ droppings	Direct contact with body fluids of infected people or animals	Respiratory droplets (close contact)	Respiratory droplets, contact with infected camels
Signs and Symptoms	Fever, muscle pain, cough, severe respiratory distress	Fever, bleeding, weakness, organ failure	Fever, dry cough, difficulty breathing	Fever, cough, shortness of breath
Diagnosis / Tests	Blood tests (ELISA, PCR)	PCR, ELISA, clinical observation	PCR, chest X-ray, blood tests	PCR, chest imaging, blood tests
Prevention / Prophylaxis	Avoid rodent contact, sanitize areas, wear masks in high-risk zones	Avoid contact with infected fluids or people, PPE use	Mask use, hygiene, isolation of infected	Hygiene, camel handling precautions, mask use
Treatment	Supportive care only, hospitalization needed	Supportive care, isolation, immediate medical attention	Supportive care, oxygen therapy	Hospital care, isolation, symptom management
Geographic Distribution	Americas (U.S., South America)	Central and West Africa, outbreaks elsewhere	Asia (China, worldwide outbreaks in 2003)	Middle East, some global cases

V. Fungal Diseases (Mycoses)

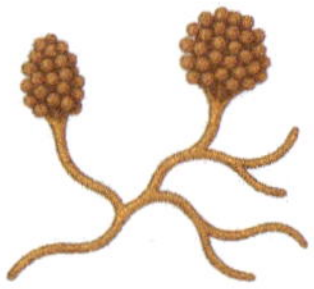

Fungal Infections: Tiny Spores, Big Impact

Fungi are incredibly important to humans—and not just in scary ways! Some of the most delicious foods we enjoy rely on fungi: edible mushrooms like champignons and shiitake, blue cheese, bread, and even beer all depend on their magical properties. And don't forget about penicillin—the world's first antibiotic—discovered from a fungus! Millions of lives have been saved thanks to these microscopic heroes.

In nature, fungi play a vital role in breaking down organic matter. Without them, the Earth would be buried under fallen trees, dead plants, and animal waste. They are the planet's recycling champions.

But, like all living organisms, some fungi have evolved to live inside or on other hosts—including us. While many fungal infections are mild and treatable, others can be serious or even life-threatening. Some of them have very long and complex names—like paracoccidioidomycosis, chromoblastomycosis, or Jorge Lobo's disease—and although rare, they highlight how diverse and adaptable fungi can be.

In this chapter, we'll focus on the most important fungal diseases that can be transmitted from animals or environments to humans. Let's explore these mysterious spores and learn how to stay safe from their invisible dangers!

Common Name of the Disease	Scientific Name	Animals or Sources Associated with the Fungus
*Histoplasmosis	*Histoplasma capsulatum*	Bird and bat droppings
Valley Fever (Coccidioidomycosis)	*Coccidioides* spp.	Soil, rodents (in arid regions)
Cryptococcosis	*Cryptococcus neoformans*	Pigeon droppings
Paracoccidioidomycosis	*Paracoccidioides brasiliensis*	Soil (associated with armadillos)
Ringworm (Dermatophytosis)	*Microsporum canis, Trichophyton* spp.	Cats, dogs, horses, cattle

*See an example of the most dangerous one below.

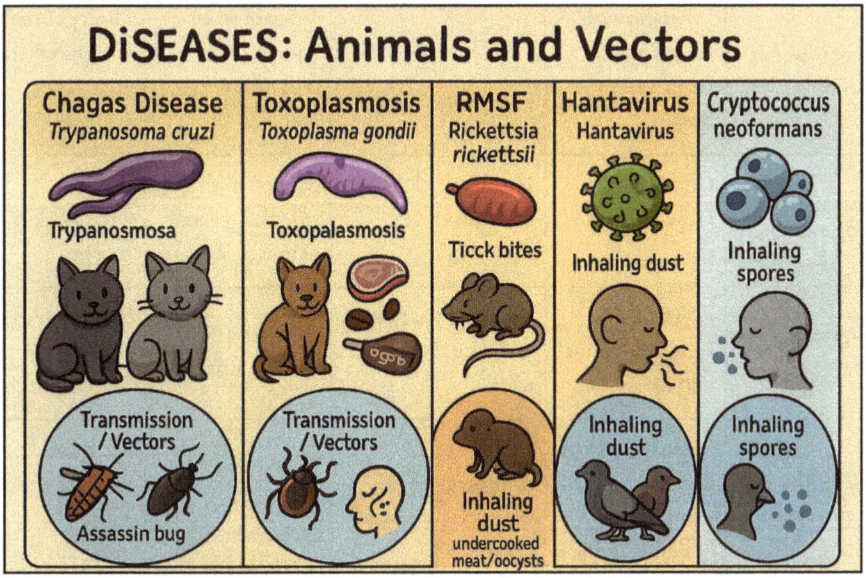

Understanding is protection!

Each animal, vector, and microorganism in this image plays a role in the transmission of diseases. By learning how these pathogens spread—and recognizing early signs and symptoms—we can take action, seek medical help when needed, and protect our families and communities.

💡 **Knowledge saves lives.**

So don't keep this to yourself—share what you learn with friends and help others stay safe too!

Silent and Persistent: Fungal Infections from the Environment and Animals

This table presents four significant fungal diseases that can affect humans, many with zoonotic or environmental links. Fungi are everywhere—in the soil, in animal waste, even in our pets' fur. While some cause mild skin issues, others can lead to life-threatening infections, especially in people with weakened immune systems. Knowing how they're transmitted and how to avoid exposure is key to staying healthy in environments where these pathogens thrive.

Characteristics	Valley Fever (Coccidioidomycosis)	Cryptococcosis	Paracoccidioidomycosis	Ringworm (Dermatophytosis)
Transmission / Vectors	Inhalation of fungal spores from soil or dust	Inhalation of spores from pigeon droppings	Inhalation of spores from contaminated soil	Direct contact with infected animals or surfaces
Signs and Symptoms	Cough, fever, fatigue, chest pain	Headache, fever, confusion, meningitis	Mouth ulcers, breathing issues, skin lesions	Itchy, red, circular skin patches
Diagnosis / Tests	Chest X-ray, serology, fungal culture	CSF analysis, India ink stain, blood tests	Serology, biopsy, imaging	Skin scrapings, Wood's lamp, fungal culture
Prevention / Prophylaxis	Avoid dusty areas, use masks in endemic zones	Avoid contact with bird droppings, wear masks in risk areas	Avoid soil exposure in endemic areas	Maintain hygiene, avoid sharing personal items
Treatment	Antifungal treatment, seek medical help	Antifungal medication, urgent medical care	Medical follow-up with antifungal therapy	Topical or oral antifungals (under medical advice)
Geographic Distribution	Southwestern U.S., Mexico, Central & South America	Worldwide, especially in urban bird zones	South America (mainly Brazil, Colombia)	Worldwide (cosmopolitan), common in warm climates

*Disease 5: Histoplasmosis

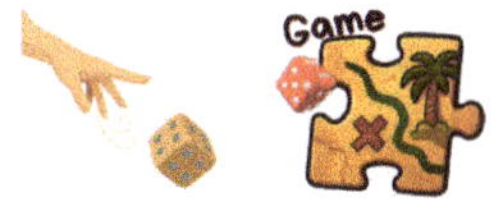

Transmission / Vectors

Histoplasmosis is caused by a fungus found in bird and bat droppings. People get infected by breathing in spores from the air—especially in caves, chicken coops, or old buildings.

Signs and Symptoms

Many people don't feel sick at all. But some may get cough, fever, chest pain, and feel very tired—just like the flu. In severe cases, it can affect the lungs for a long time or even spread to other organs.

Diagnosis / Tests

Doctors use blood tests, urine tests, or chest X-rays to detect the fungus or signs of lung infection.

Prevention / Prophylaxis

Avoid areas with lots of bat or bird droppings, especially dusty places. Wear a mask if working in barns, caves, or cleaning old buildings. Don't stir up the dust!

Treatment

Mild cases usually go away on their own. Severe cases are treated with antifungal medicines taken for weeks or months.

Geographic Distribution

Histoplasmosis is found in many parts of the world—especially in the Americas, including the Amazon, the Ohio and Mississippi River Valleys in the U.S., and parts of Asia and Africa.

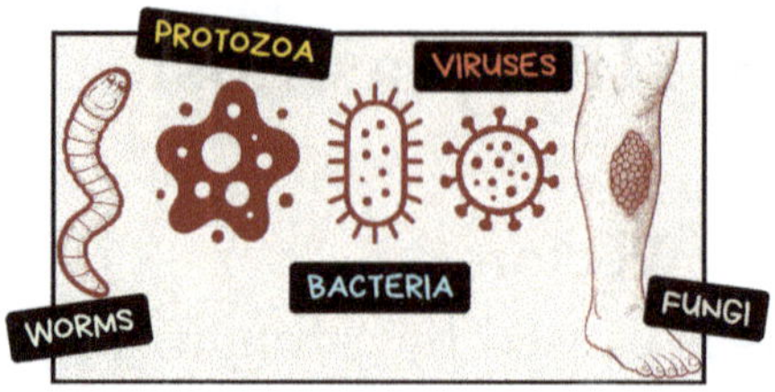

Here we have the five major groups of pathogens: worms, protozoa, bacteria, viruses, and fungi. They're all around us—so stay alert, learn, enjoy this book, and have fun. But watch out... parasites are sneaky!

This list highlights the vital role that wildlife plays in maintaining the life cycles of parasites and pathogens.

Many wild animals, from small rodents to large mammals, unknowingly carry, transport, or contribute to the transmission of microorganisms—whether to other animals, to vectors like insects and ticks, or even to humans. They are not villains; they are part of the intricate balance of ecosystems, shaped over millions of years.

That's why conservation and responsible human interaction with nature are essential. As we encroach further into forests, alter habitats, and disrupt natural cycles, we increase the chances of zoonotic spillovers—when diseases jump from animals to humans.

But here's the key message: the responsibility for prevention lies with us. Through education, hygiene, avoiding unnecessary contact with wildlife, keeping our domestic animals healthy, and supporting ecological balance, we can dramatically reduce the risk of infections.

By staying informed and alert, we not only protect ourselves and our communities—we also help preserve the incredible biodiversity of our planet.

The Parasite Dice Game I

Roll the dice and start your parasite adventure!
Use a real die or a dice app on your phone to play!
First, roll the die once to choose which disease you'll face.
Then, roll again to select one of its key characteristics (like how it spreads or how to prevent it!).
Got it right? Score 10 points!
Got it wrong? Pass the die to the next player.
Who will be the best Parasite Hunter? Let the battle of brains and biology begin!

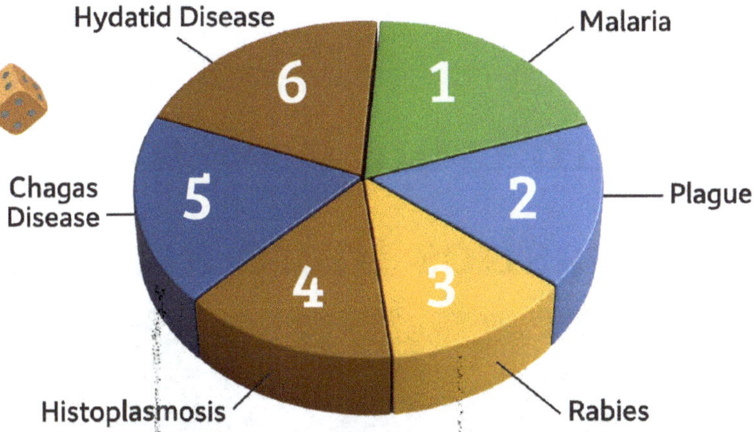

Key Characteristics to Know:

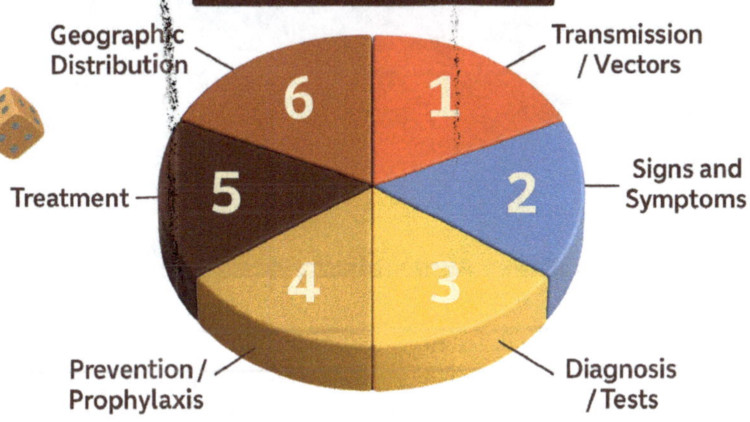

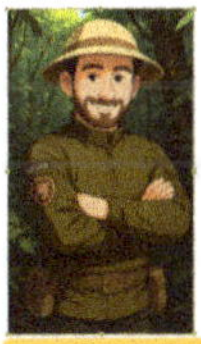

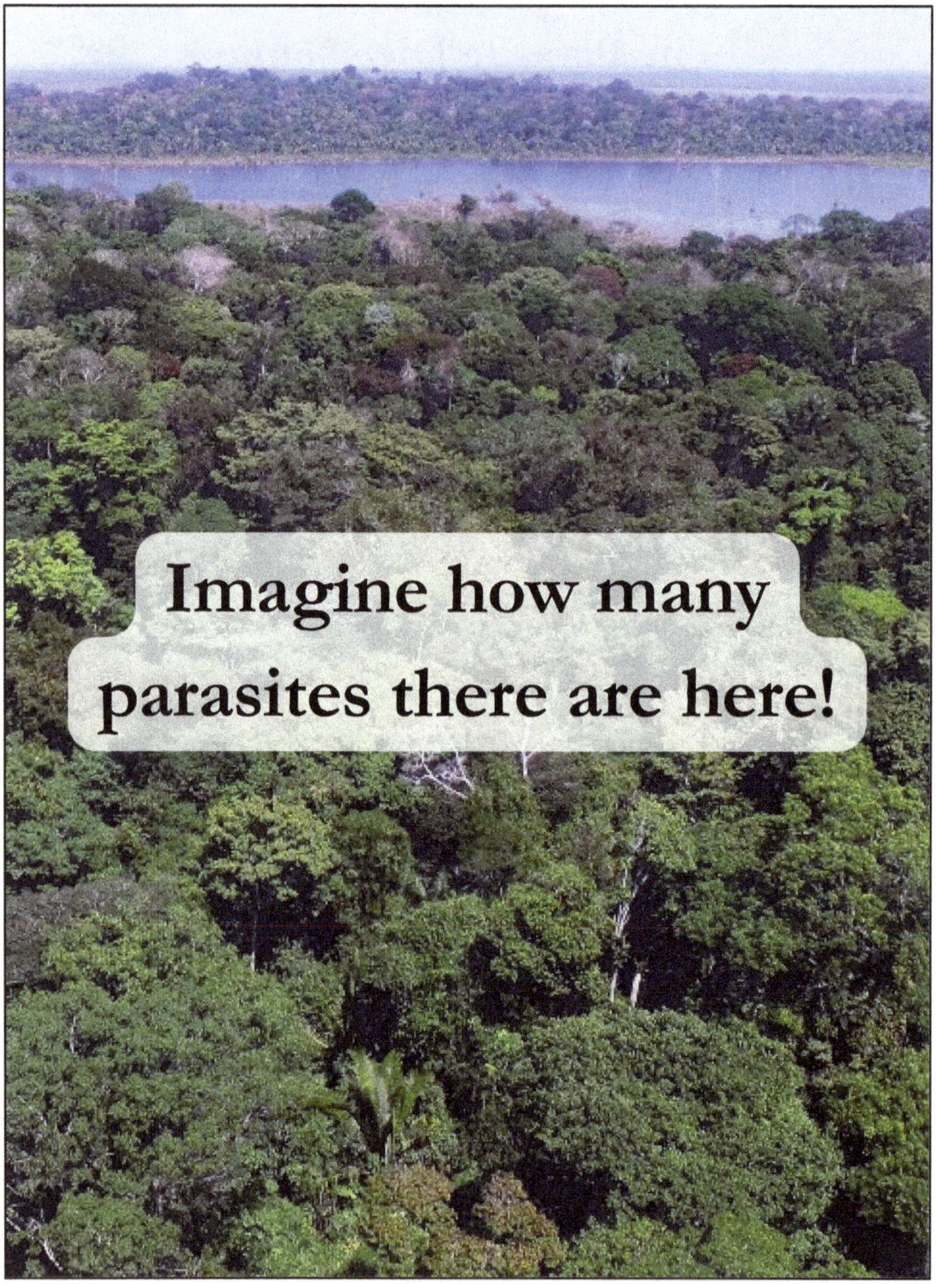

Hidden Carriers of the Wild – In this lush Amazonian landscape, located in the Samuel Ecological Station forest in Candeias do Jamari, about 56 miles (90 km) from the capital Porto Velho, which animals might be silently carrying parasites and pathogens?
Before venturing into environments like this, stop and think: could you walk out carrying more than just memories—perhaps a hidden parasite?

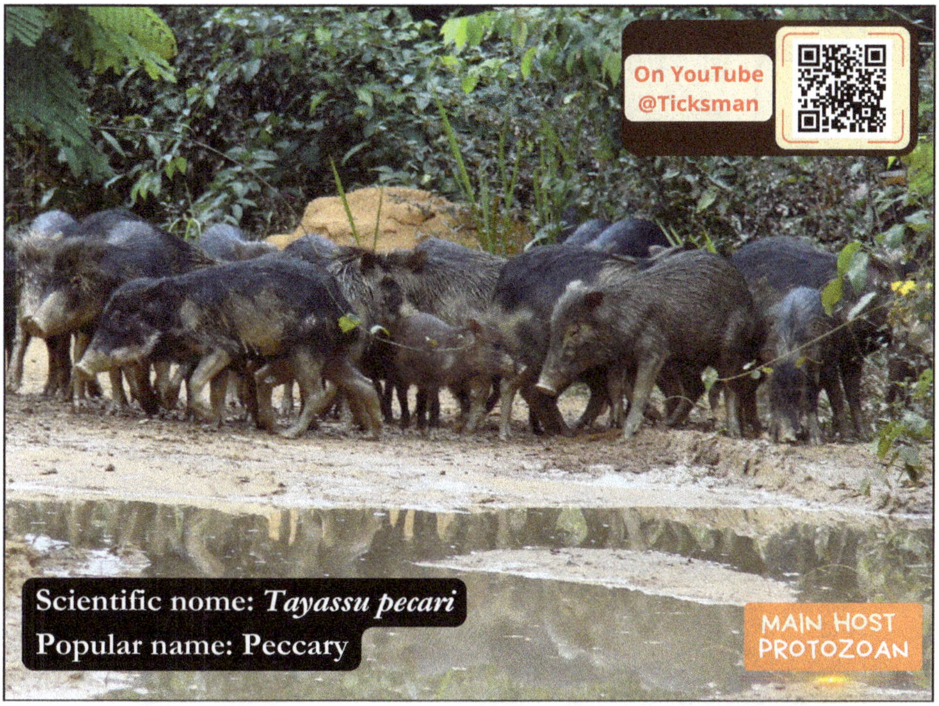
On YouTube
@Ticksman
Scientific nome: Tayassu pecari
Popular name: Peccary
MAIN HOST
PROTOZOAN

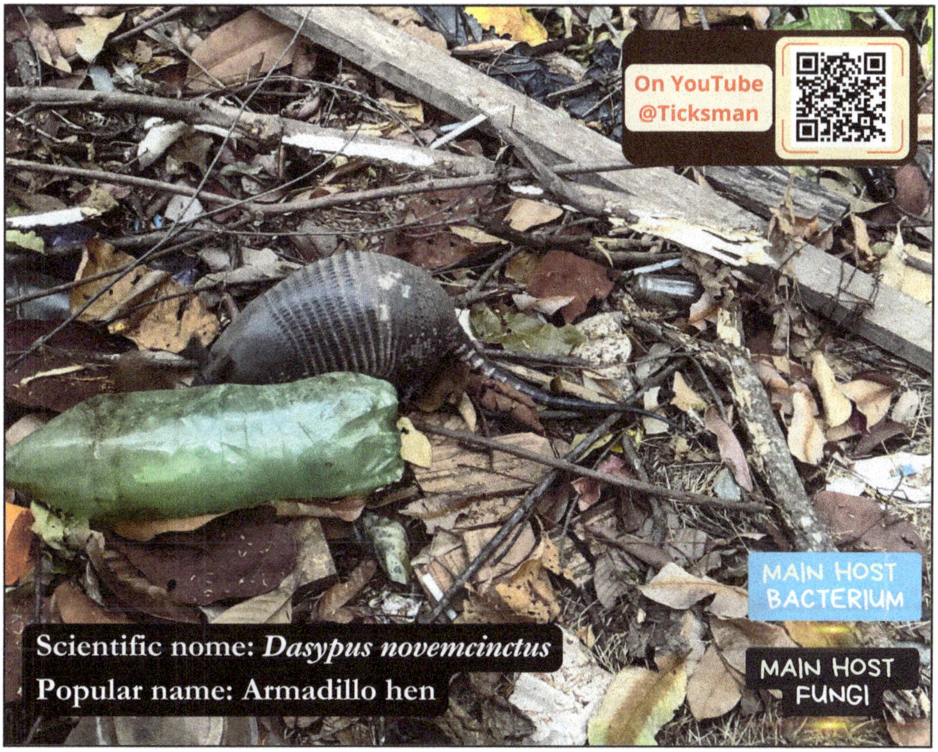
On YouTube
@Ticksman
MAIN HOST
BACTERIUM
Scientific nome: Dasypus novemcinctus
Popular name: Armadillo hen
MAIN HOST
FUNGI

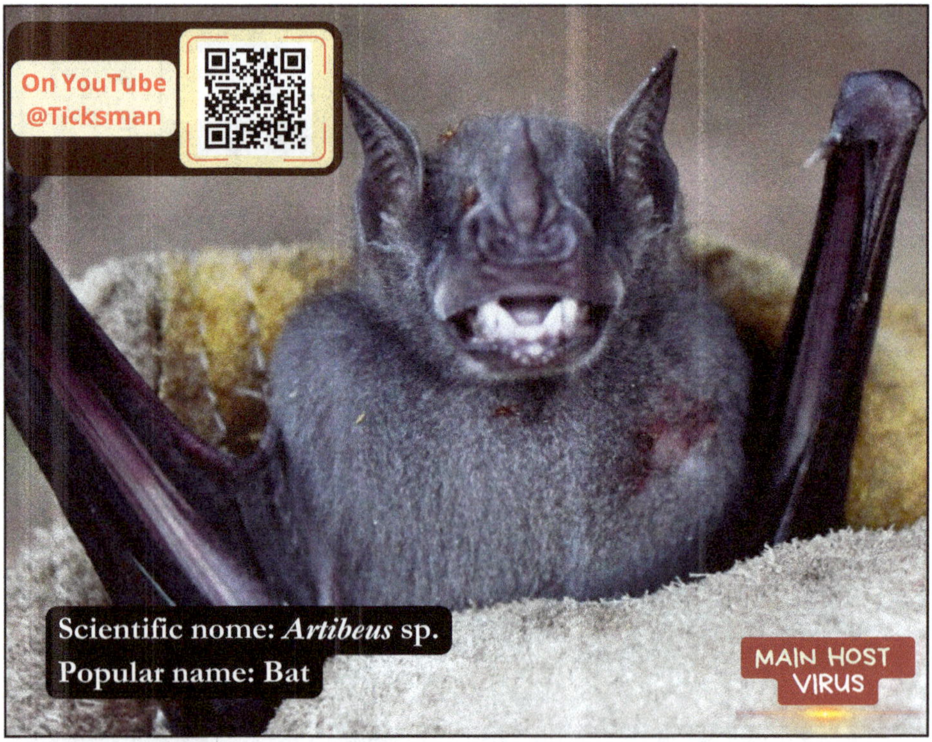
On YouTube
@Ticksman
Scientific nome: *Artibeus* sp.
Popular name: Bat
MAIN HOST
VIRUS

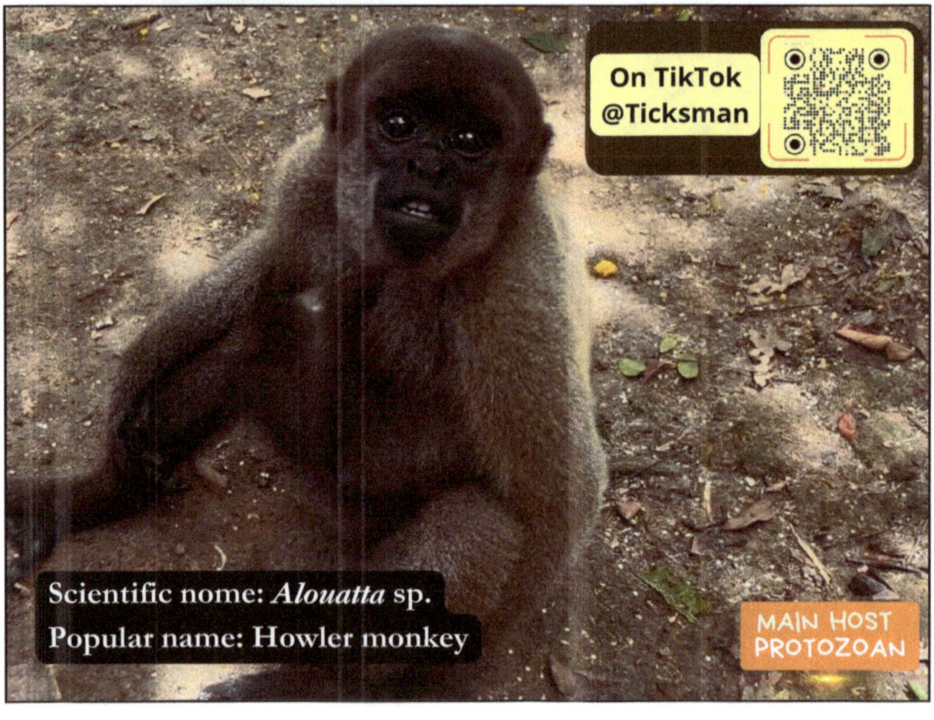
On TikTok
@Ticksman
Scientific nome: *Alouatta* sp.
Popular name: Howler monkey
MAIN HOST
PROTOZOAN

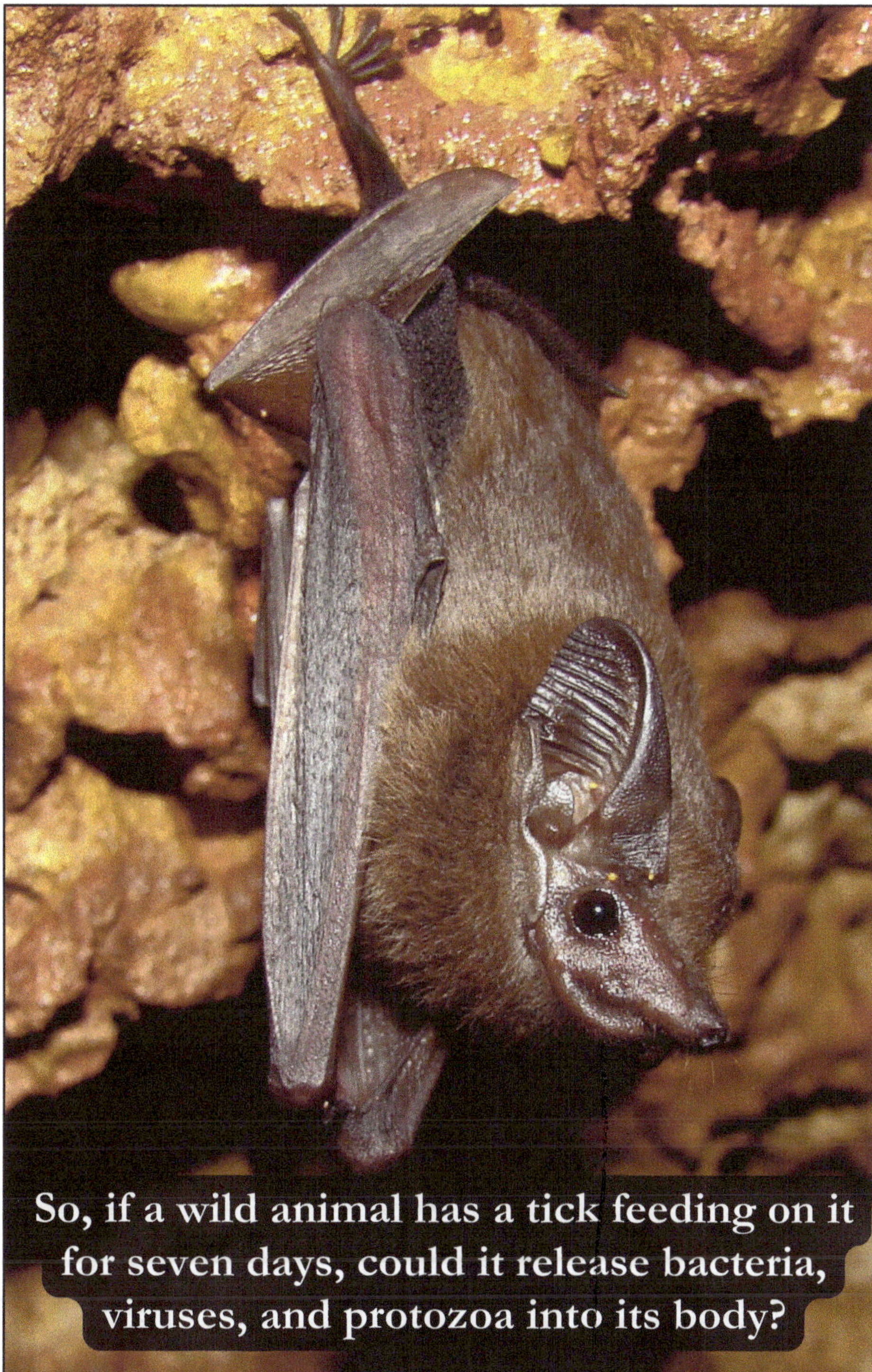
So, if a wild animal has a tick feeding on it
for seven days, could it release bacteria,
viruses, and protozoa into its body?

Now, let's take a closer look. In the image, you can see tick nymphs, fully engorged with blood after seven days of continuous feeding on the ear of an agouti (*Dasyprocta* spp.). During this prolonged attachment, something critical happens: if the tick is already infected with a microorganism—whether a bacterium, virus, or protozoan—it will transmit the pathogen to the agouti through its saliva.

But the transmission works both ways. If the agouti is already carrying a different microorganism in its bloodstream, the feeding tick can ingest the pathogen along with the blood. Once the tick completes its meal, it will drop to the ground, undergo metamorphosis into its adult stage, and seek a new host. If that next host happens to be a human, the infected tick can transmit the acquired pathogen, potentially causing a parasitic disease.

This intricate exchange between host and parasite is what makes ticks such efficient vectors of disease, silently bridging the gap between wildlife, domestic animals, and humans in tropical ecosystems.

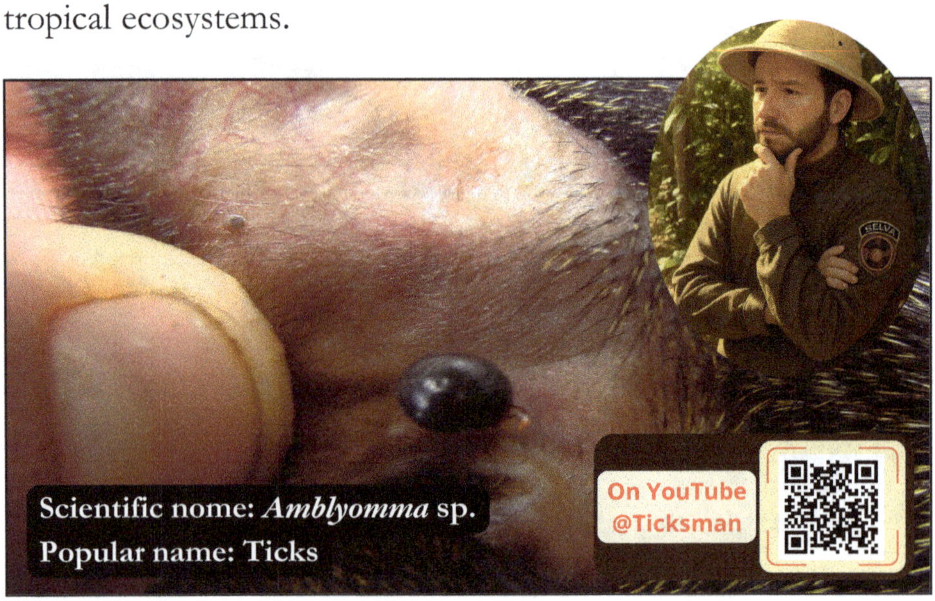

Scientific nome: *Amblyomma* sp.
Popular name: Ticks

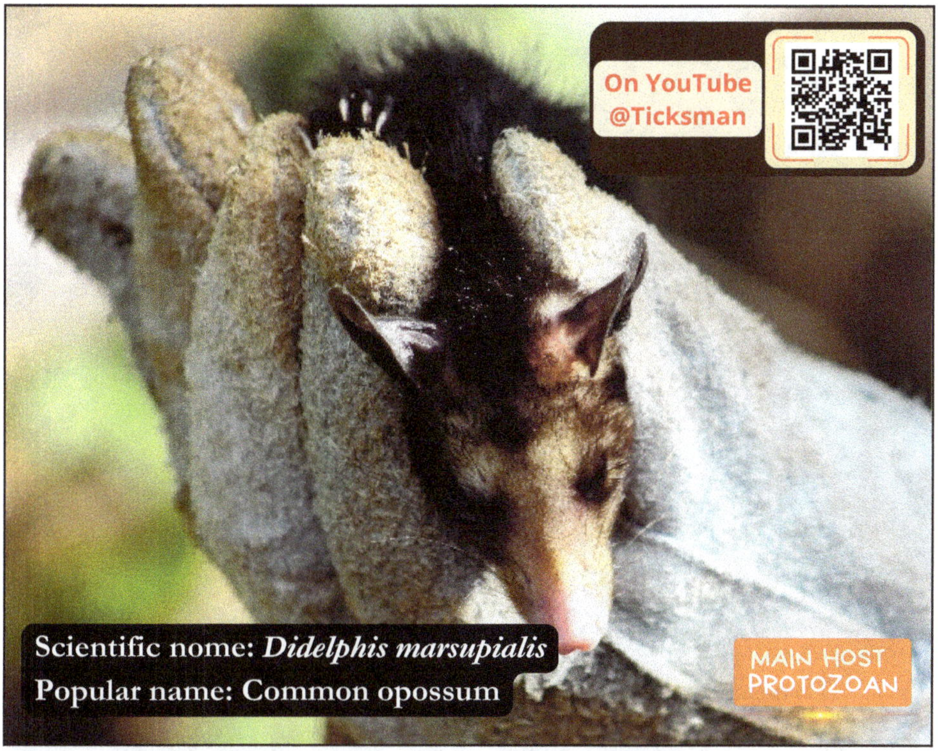
On YouTube
@Ticksman
Scientific nome: *Didelphis marsupialis*
Popular name: Common opossum
MAIN HOST
PROTOZOAN

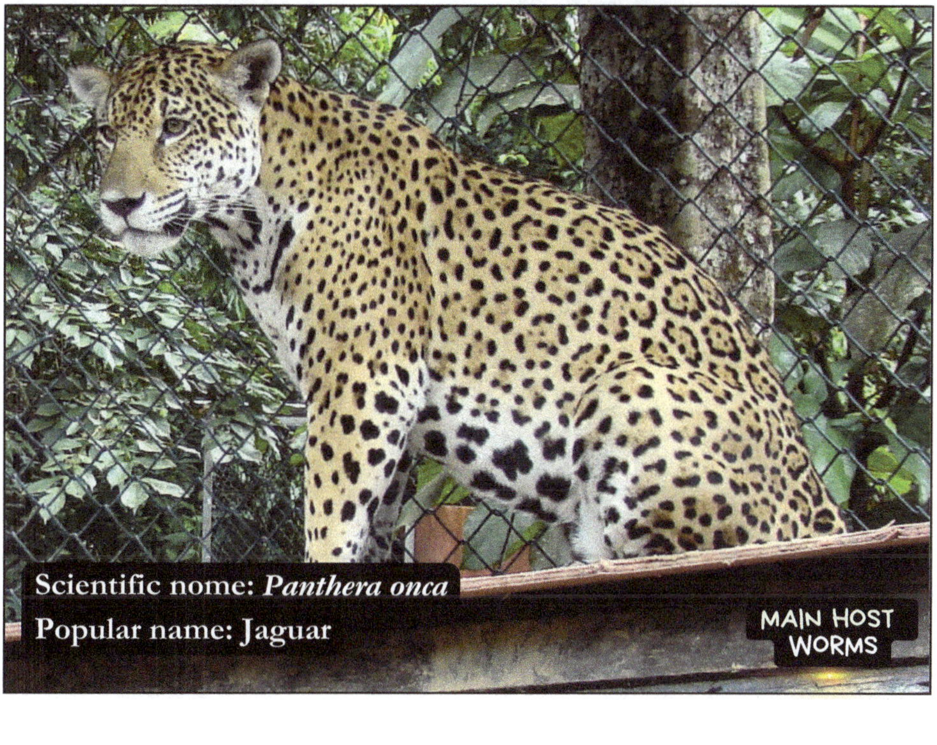
Scientific nome: *Panthera onca*
Popular name: Jaguar
MAIN HOST
WORMS

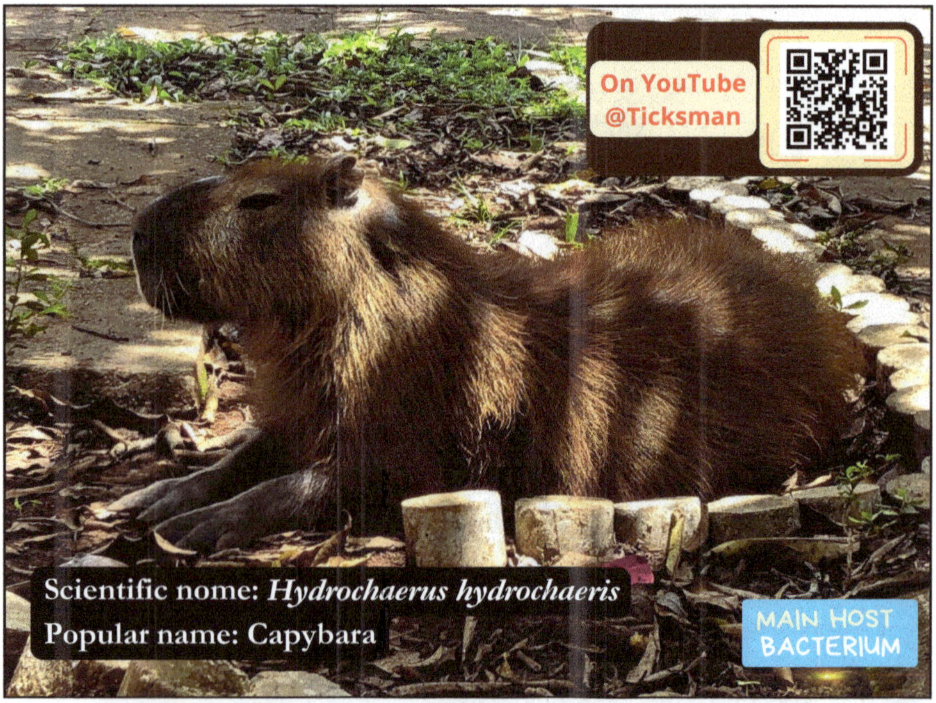
On YouTube
@Ticksman
Scientific nome: *Hydrochaerus hydrochaeris*
Popular name: Capybara
MAIN HOST
BACTERIUM

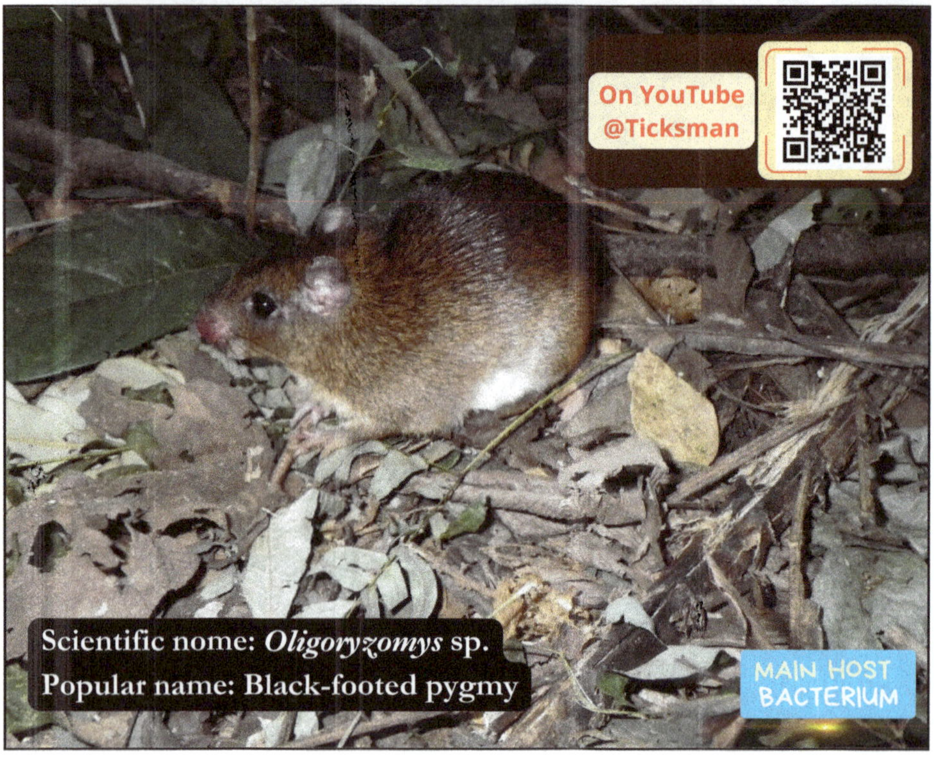
On YouTube
@Ticksman
Scientific nome: *Oligoryzomys* sp.
Popular name: Black-footed pygmy
MAIN HOST
BACTERIUM

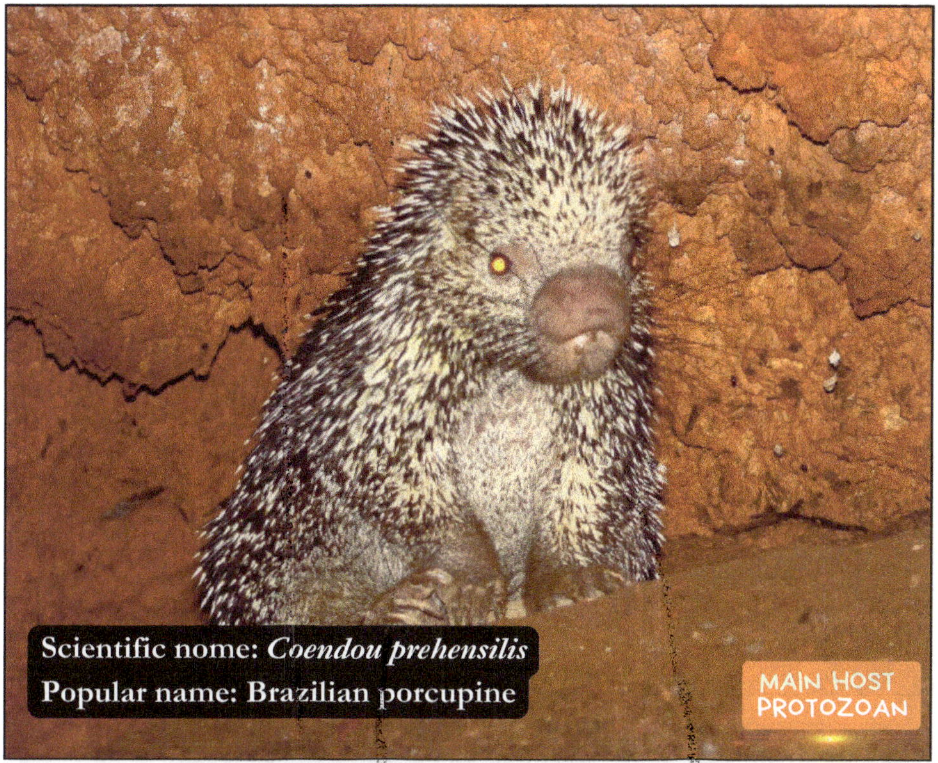
Scientific nome: *Coendou prehensilis*
Popular name: Brazilian porcupine
MAIN HOST
PROTOZOAN

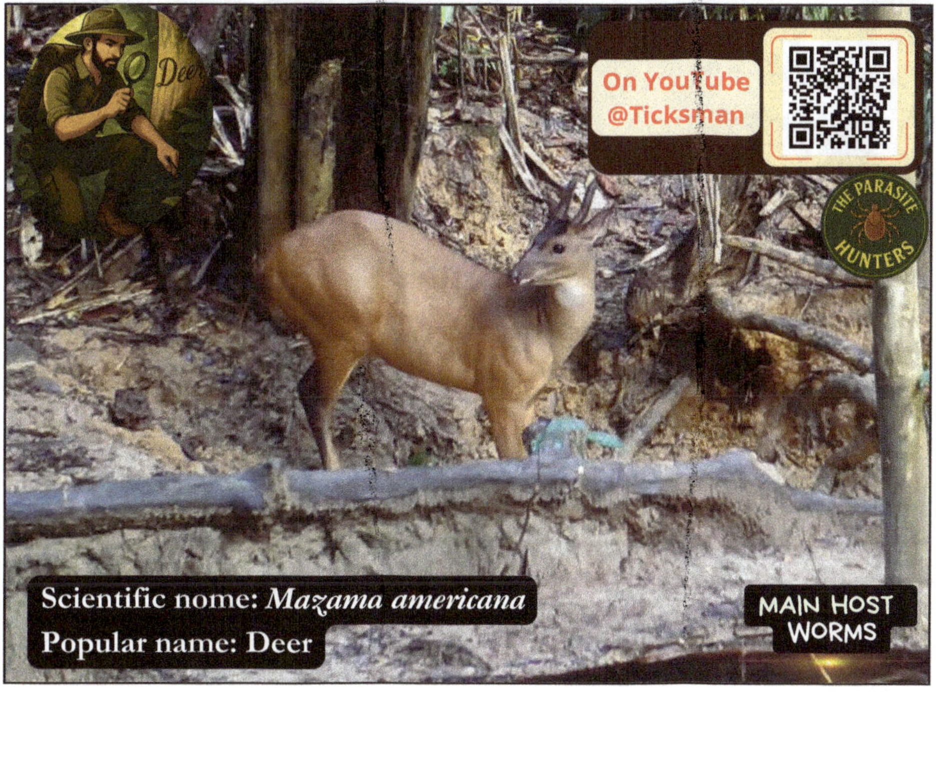
On YouTube
@Ticksman
THE PARASITE HUNTERS
Scientific nome: *Mazama americana*
Popular name: Deer
MAIN HOST
WORMS

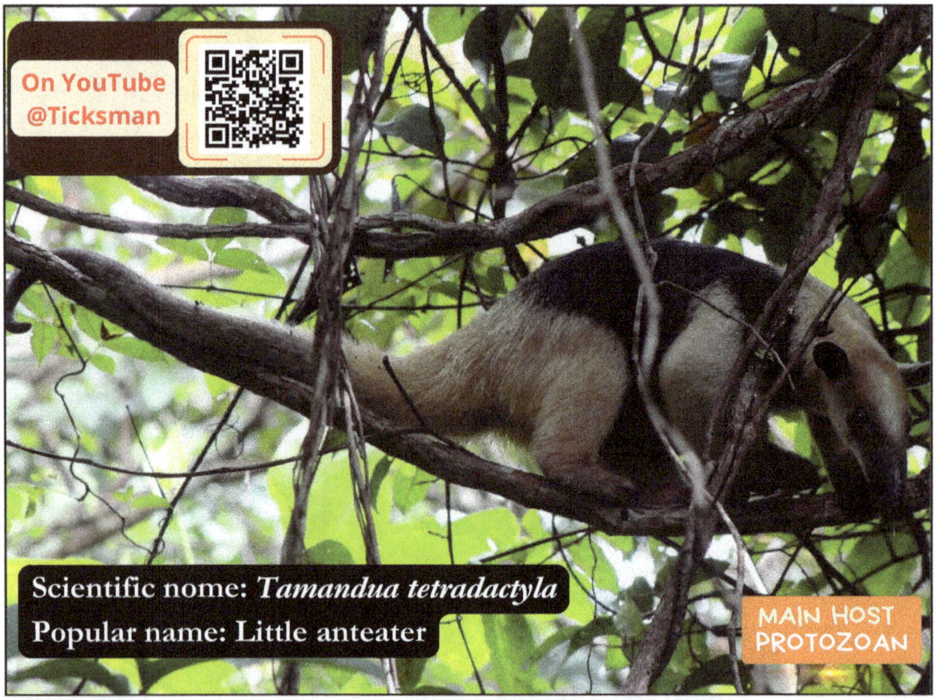
On YouTube
@Ticksman
Scientific nome: *Tamandua tetradactyla*
Popular name: Little anteater
MAIN HOST
PROTOZOAN

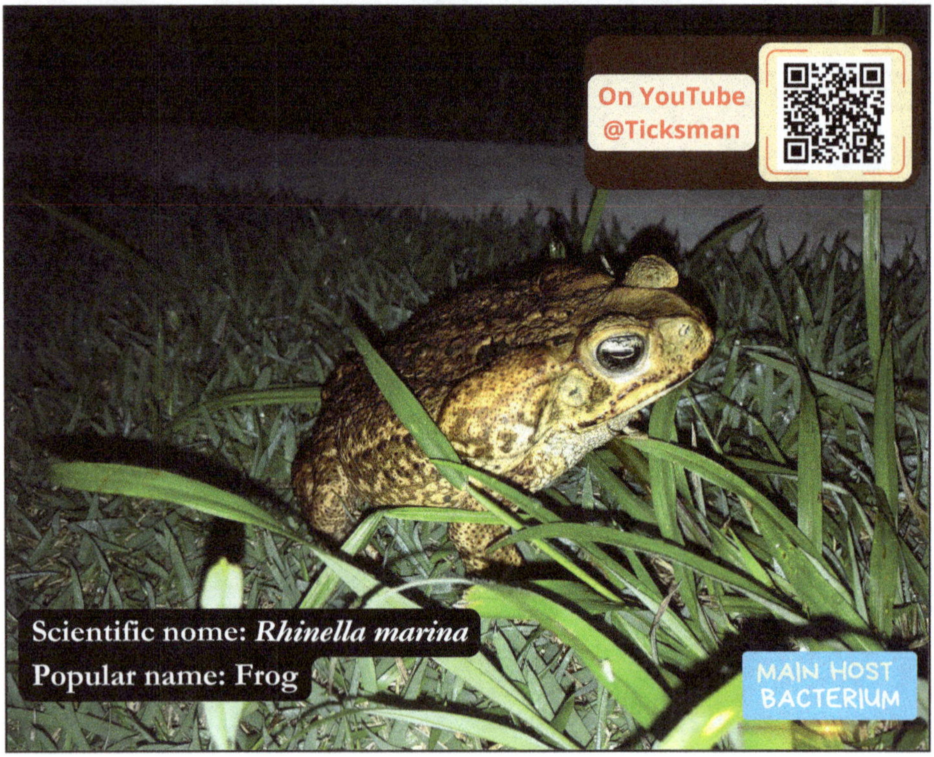
On YouTube
@Ticksman
Scientific nome: *Rhinella marina*
Popular name: Frog
MAIN HOST
BACTERIUM

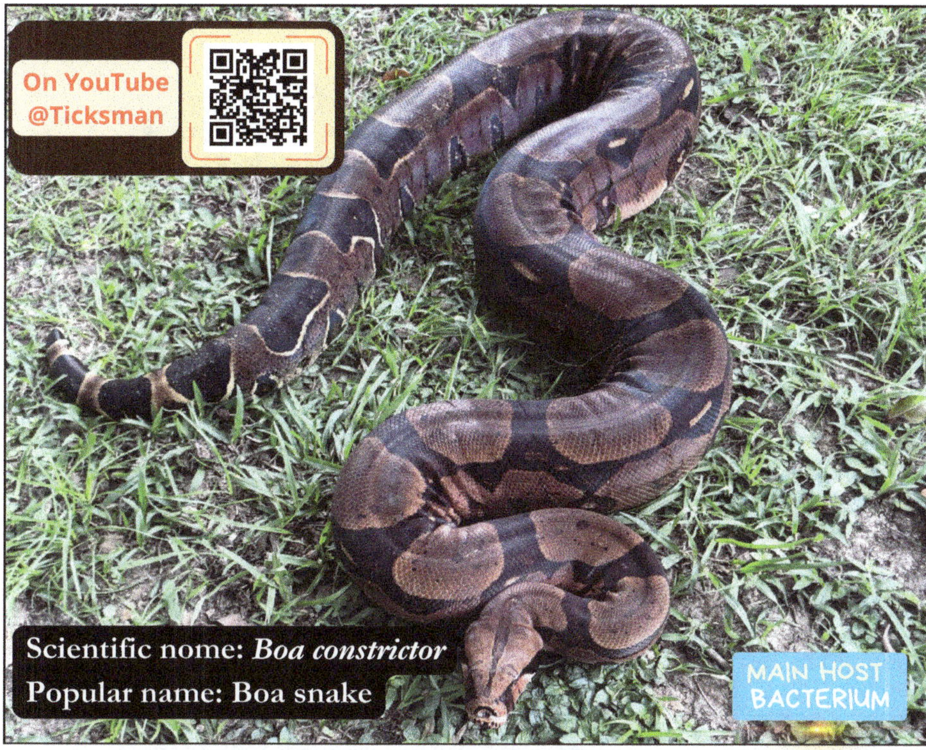
On YouTube
@Ticksman
Scientific nome: *Boa constrictor*
Popular name: Boa snake
MAIN HOST
BACTERIUM

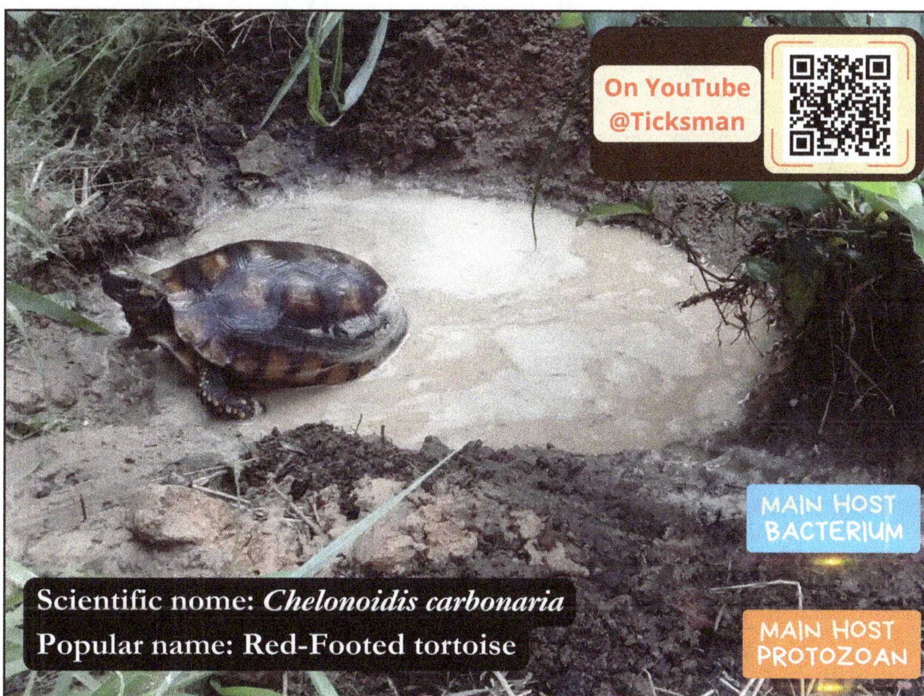
On YouTube
@Ticksman
MAIN HOST
BACTERIUM
Scientific nome: *Chelonoidis carbonaria*
Popular name: Red-Footed tortoise
MAIN HOST
PROTOZOAN

Wild Animals & Their Main Pathogen Groups

This table highlights a selection of important zoonotic diseases linked to wild animals, organized by the main pathogen groups—worms, protozoa, bacteria, viruses, and fungi. While many other diseases can be associated with each species, the ones shown here were chosen for their relevance and known impact. Remember: our planet is vast, and what's common in one region may be rare or unknown in another.

Animal	Main Pathogen Group	Example of Related Disease
Wild pig (Cateto - peccary)	**Protozoa**	*Trypanosoma cruzi* – Chagas Disease
Porcupine	**Protozoa**	*Leishmania* spp. – Potential wild reservoir
Tamandua (lesser anteater)	**Protozoa**	*Trypanosoma cruzi* – Chagas Disease
Howler monkey	**Protozoa**	*Plasmodium* spp. – Simian Malaria
Opossum (*Didelphis* spp.)	**Protozoa**	*Trypanosoma cruzi* – Chagas Disease
Boa constrictor	**Bacteria**	*Salmonella* spp.
Capybara	**Bacteria**	*Rickettsia rickettsii* – Brazilian Spotted Fever
Wild rodent	**Bacteria**	*Leptospira* spp., *Yersinia pestis* – Plague
Yellow-footed tortoise	**Bacteria**	*Salmonella* spp. and other enterobacteria
Cane toad (*Rhinella marina*)	**Bacteria / Fungi**	Dermatophytes, *Salmonella* spp.
Jaguar	**Worms**	*Toxocara* spp., *Ancylostoma* spp.
Deer (Amazonian)	**Worms**	*Fasciola hepatica, Taenia* spp.
Bat	**Viruses**	Rabies virus, *Ebolavirus, Marburg virus*
Armadillo	**Fungi**	*Paracoccidioides brasiliensis* – Paracoccidioidomycosis

IMPORTANT REMINDER:

LOVE AND PROTECT, DON'T BLAME!

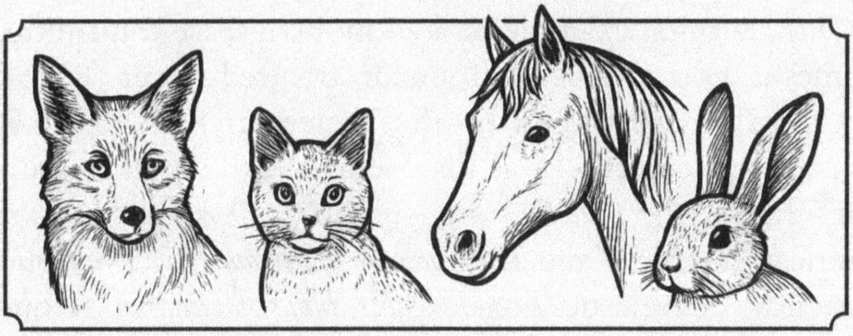

Although animals can host or carry parasites and diseases, they don't know this—they have no idea they might be transmitting anything.

If you have a pet—wild or domestic—remember: with proper care, your animal will stay healthy, and so will your family.

THE SOLUTION IS NOT FEAR OR ABANDONMENT, BUT KNOWLEDGE AND RESPONSIBILITY.

Help spread this message: animals are not the enemy. They need our care, not our rejection.

Urban & Domestic Hosts: Silent Carriers Among Us

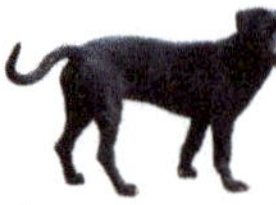

Our homes and farms are filled with animals that provide companionship, work, and sustenance. However, these same beloved pets and livestock can silently harbor parasites and pathogens that pose serious health risks to both animals and humans. From dogs and cats to chickens, horses, cattle, and pigs, every domestic animal has the potential to become a host for parasites if proper care is not maintained.

One alarming example of a zoonotic disease transmitted by a domestic host is Rocky Mountain Spotted Fever (RMSF) in the United States, caused by the bacterium *Rickettsia rickettsii.* The primary vectors of this disease in North America are ticks from the genus *Dermacentor*—notably *Dermacentor variabilis* (American dog tick) and *Dermacentor andersoni* (Rocky Mountain wood tick). Domestic dogs (*Canis lupus familiaris*) frequently serve as hosts for these ticks, bringing them into close contact with humans and increasing the risk of disease transmission.

In Brazil, a similar scenario occurs with Brazilian Spotted Fever (BSF), also caused by *Rickettsia rickettsii* but transmitted primarily by the carrapato-estrela (*Amblyomma sculptum*), which commonly infests horses.

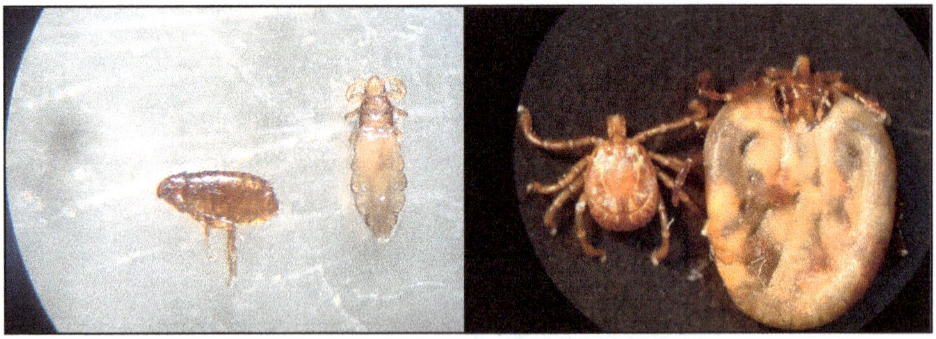

A flea, a louse and a couple of ticks, "Vector" transmitters of these pathogens to humans.

Humans are at risk when they come into contact with these infected ticks, particularly in rural or forested areas where horses serve as reservoirs.

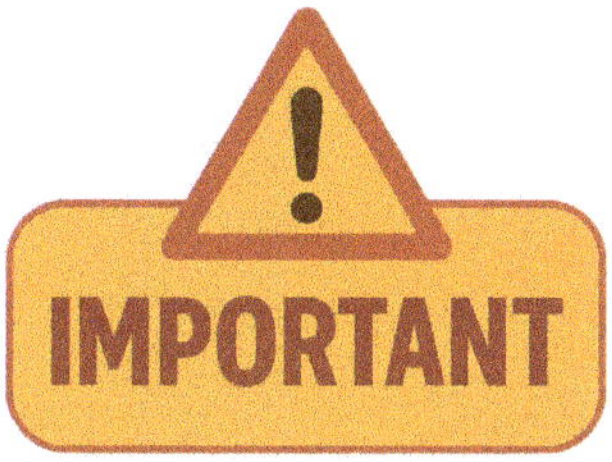

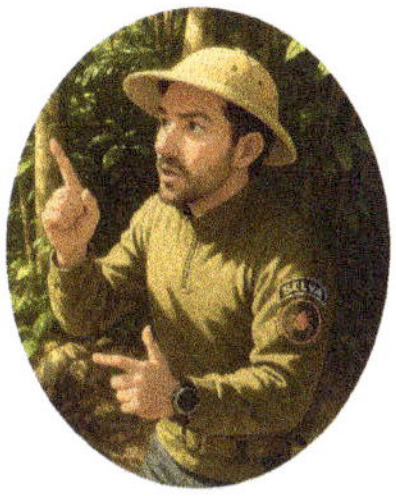

The Importance of Veterinary Care & Preventive Measures

Regular veterinary check-ups and adherence to vaccination schedules are crucial for keeping domestic animals healthy and preventing the spread of diseases. Many infectious diseases that affect livestock and pets can be prevented through proper immunization, parasite control, and hygiene practices.

Vaccination: A Lifesaving Necessity

Vaccinating domestic animals is not just about protecting them—it also safeguards human health. Diseases like rabies, leptospirosis, and brucellosis can be transmitted from animals to humans, and proper immunization is the most effective way to prevent outbreaks.

For dogs, core vaccines include those for rabies, canine parvovirus, distemper, and hepatitis. Farm animals, such as cattle, pigs, and horses, also require specific vaccines against diseases that could devastate both livestock populations and human health.

Deworming: Eliminating Internal Threats

Another essential aspect of preventive care is regular deworming. Domestic and farm animals frequently harbor intestinal parasites that can affect their health and potentially be transmitted to humans. Some of the most common zoonotic worms include:

- **Dogs & Cats:** *Toxocara canis, Toxocara cati* (which cause visceral and ocular larva migrans in humans) and *Ancylostoma* spp. (hookworms, responsible for cutaneous larva migrans).
- **Cattle & Pigs:** *Taenia saginata* (beef tapeworm) and *Taenia solium* (pork tapeworm, which can cause neurocysticercosis in humans).
- **Horses:** *Strongylus* spp. (large strongyles) and *Parascaris equorum* (roundworms affecting foals and young horses).
- **Chickens & Birds:** *Ascaridia* spp. (roundworms) and *Capillaria* spp. (capillary worms).

Deworming protocols vary by species, age, and environment, but routine treatment is fundamental to preventing infections in both animals and their human caretakers.

The Hidden Danger of External Parasites

Beyond internal worms, external parasites, such as ticks, fleas, and mites, also pose significant threats.

In addition to carrying deadly bacteria like *Rickettsia* spp., ticks are vectors for several other pathogens, including *Borrelia burgdorferi* (causing Lyme disease) and *Babesia* spp. (responsible for babesiosis).

Dogs, for example, can suffer from canine ehrlichiosis and anaplasmosis, two tick-borne diseases caused by *Ehrlichia canis* and *Anaplasma platys*, respectively.

Another devastating parasitic disease affecting dogs is canine leishmaniasis, caused by *Leishmania infantum* and transmitted by sandflies (*Lutzomyia longipalpis* in the Americas).

The disease often manifests as severe skin lesions, particularly around the nose, ears, and eyes, as well as systemic organ damage. Infected dogs act as reservoirs for the parasite, which can then be transmitted to humans, making proper prevention (such as insect repellent collars and vaccination) essential.

A Shared Responsibility

Whether we live in urban areas or rural settings, our responsibility as pet owners and animal caretakers goes beyond just providing food and shelter. Regular veterinary visits, strict parasite control, and up-to-date vaccinations are crucial steps in ensuring the well-being of domestic animals and preventing the transmission of zoonotic diseases.

By taking preventive measures, we not only protect our beloved pets and livestock but also create a healthier environment for ourselves, our families, and our communities.

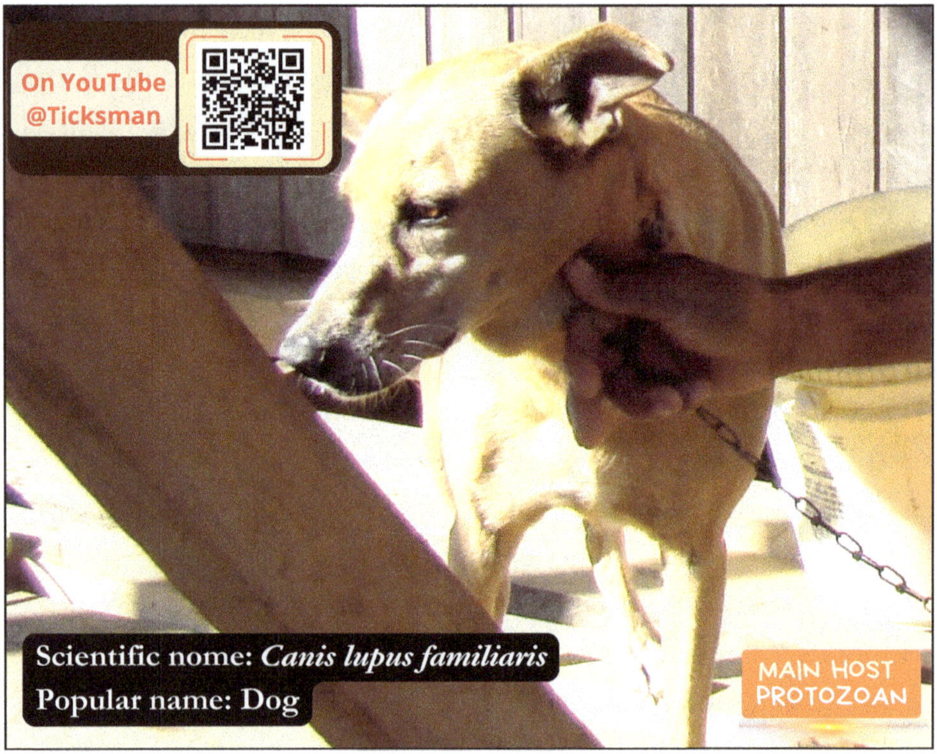
On YouTube
@Ticksman
Scientific nome: *Canis lupus familiaris*
Popular name: Dog
MAIN HOST
PROTOZOAN

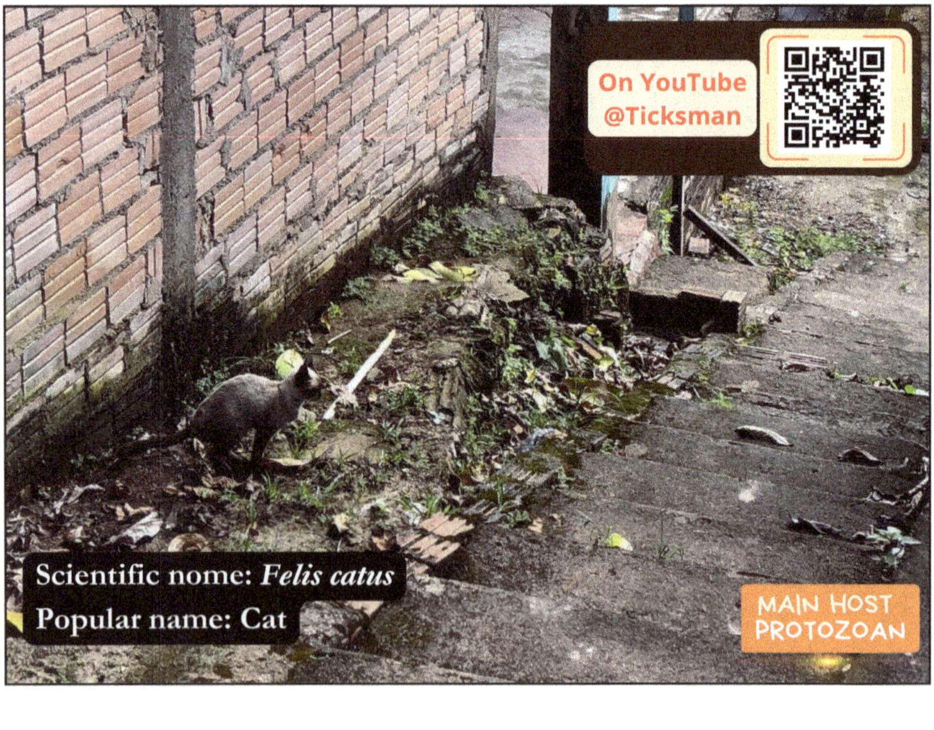
On YouTube
@Ticksman
Scientific nome: *Felis catus*
Popular name: Cat
MAIN HOST
PROTOZOAN

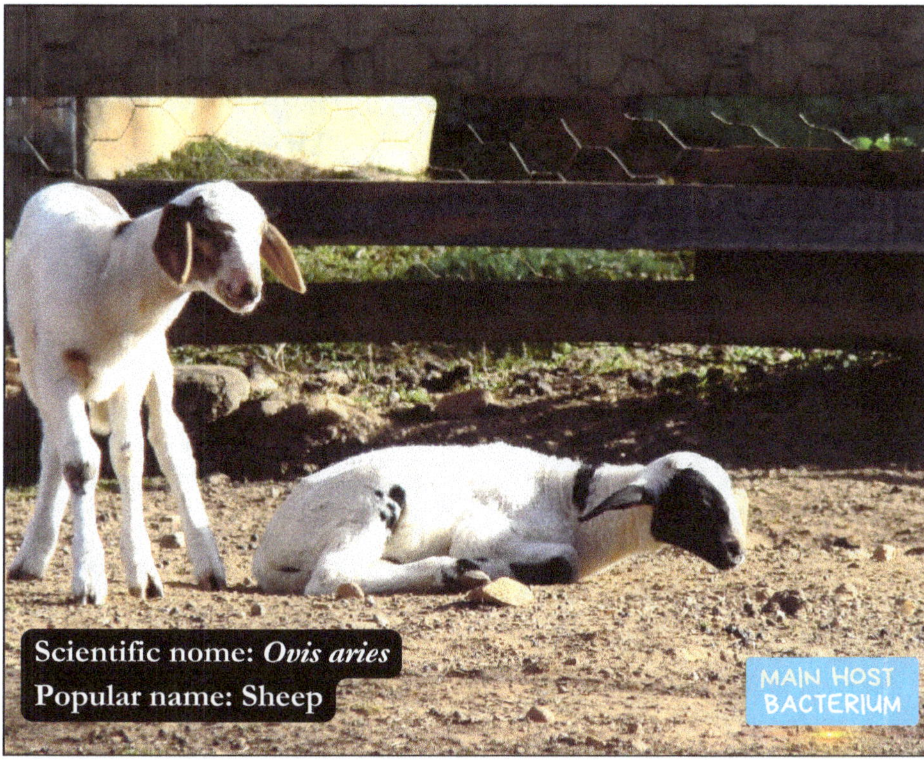
Scientific nome: *Ovis aries*
Popular name: Sheep
MAIN HOST
BACTERIUM

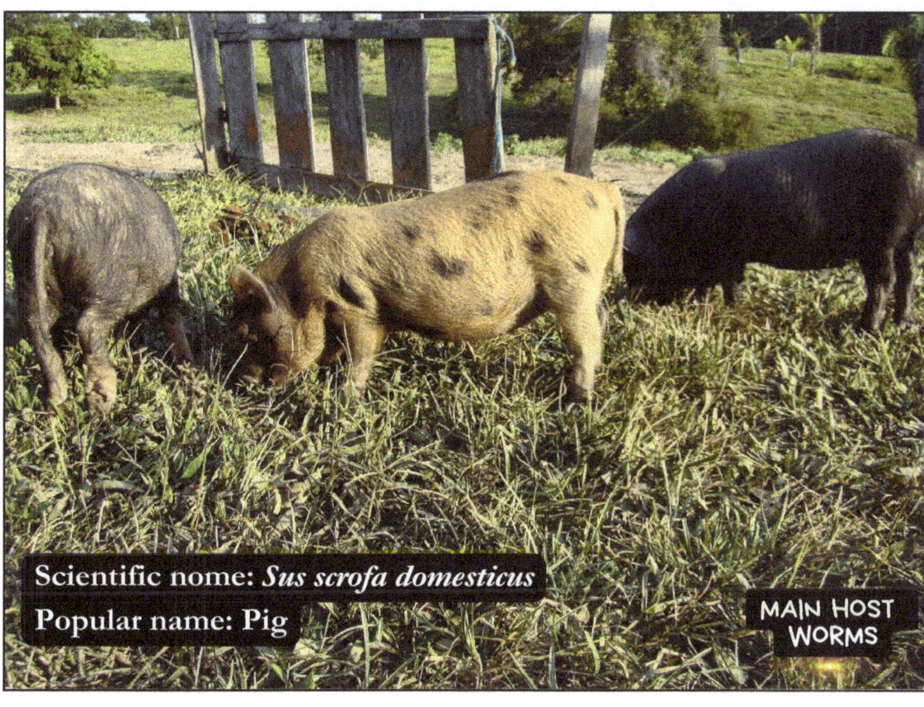
Scientific nome: *Sus scrofa domesticus*
Popular name: Pig
MAIN HOST
WORMS

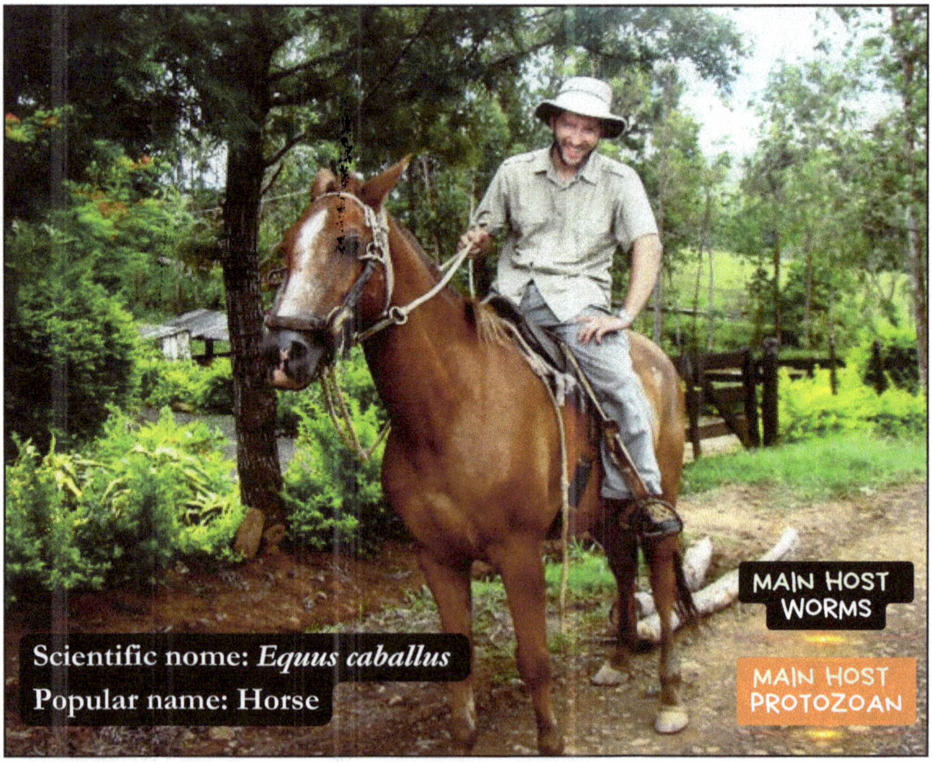
MAIN HOST
WORMS
MAIN HOST
PROTOZOAN
Scientific nome: *Equus caballus*
Popular name: Horse

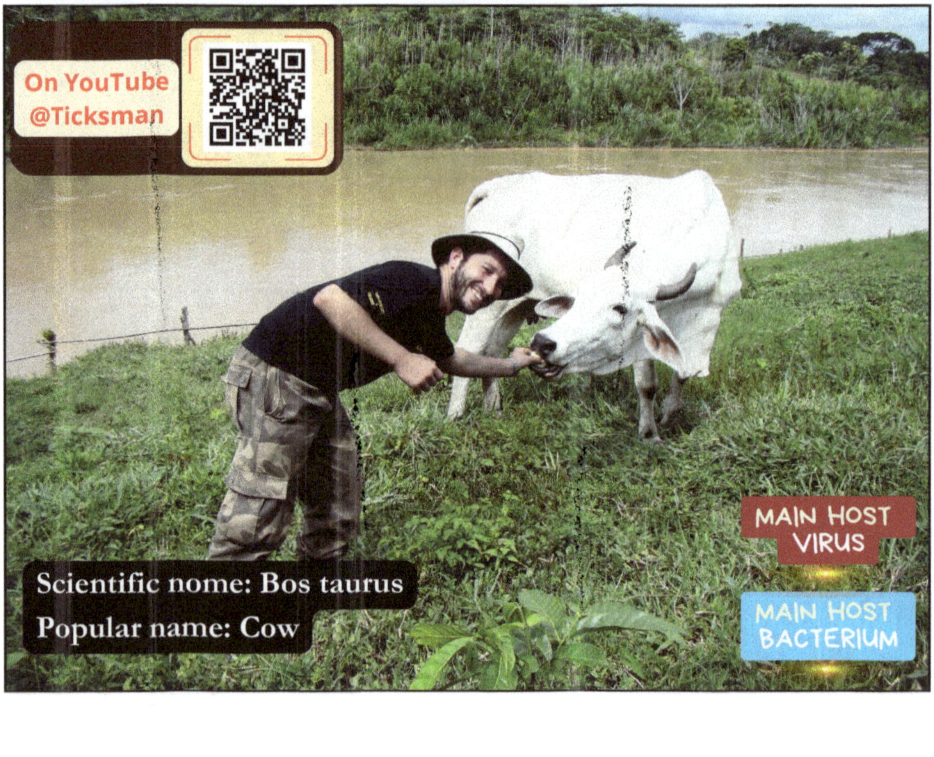
On YouTube
@Ticksman
MAIN HOST
VIRUS
MAIN HOST
BACTERIUM
Scientific nome: Bos taurus
Popular name: Cow

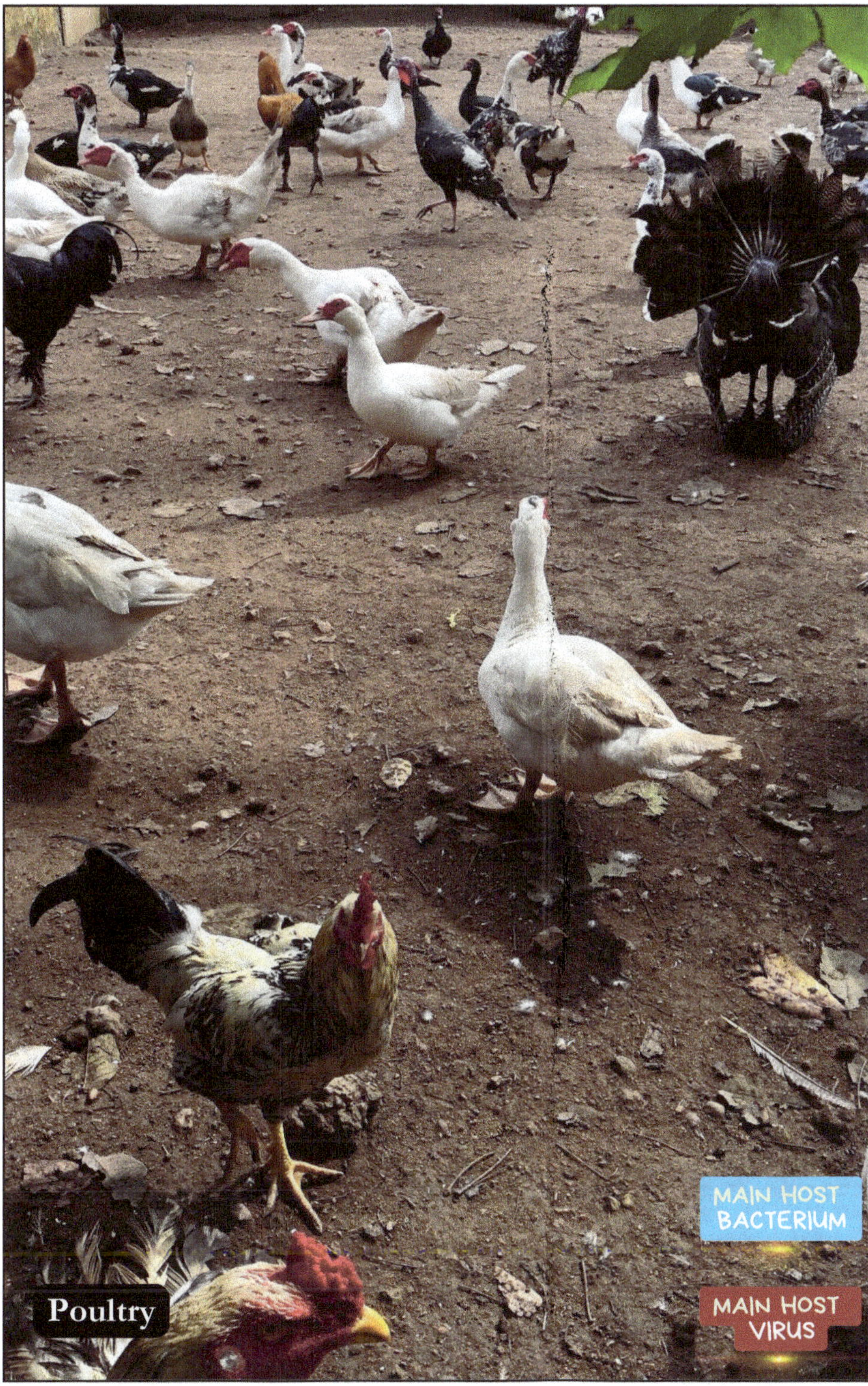
MAIN HOST
BACTERIUM
MAIN HOST
VIRUS
Poultry

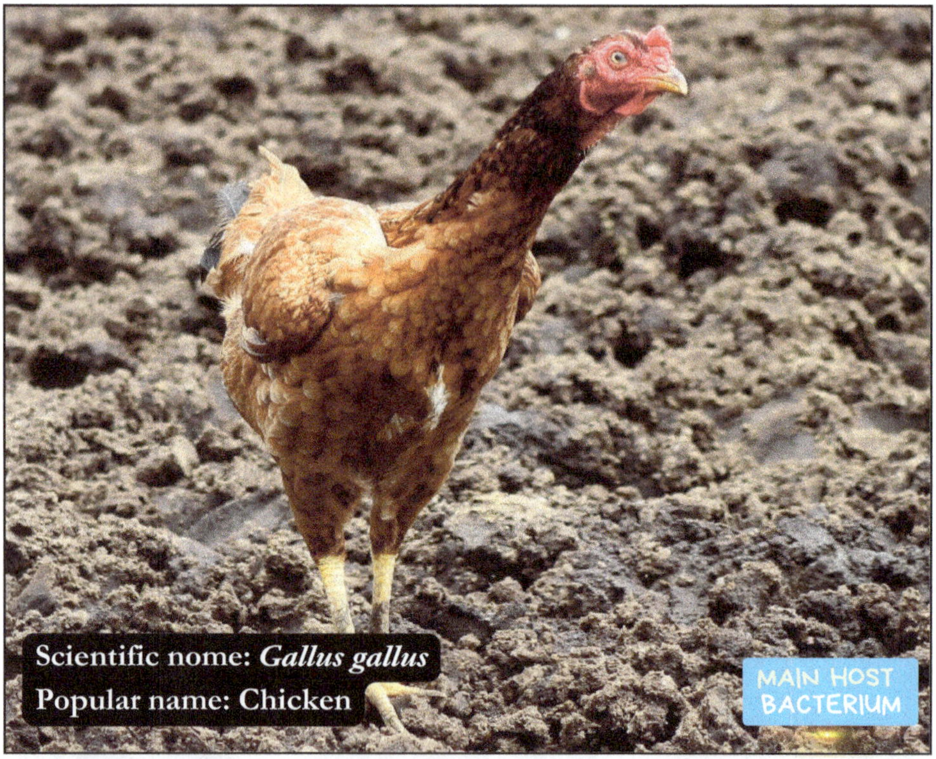
Scientific nome: *Gallus gallus*
Popular name: Chicken
MAIN HOST
BACTERIUM

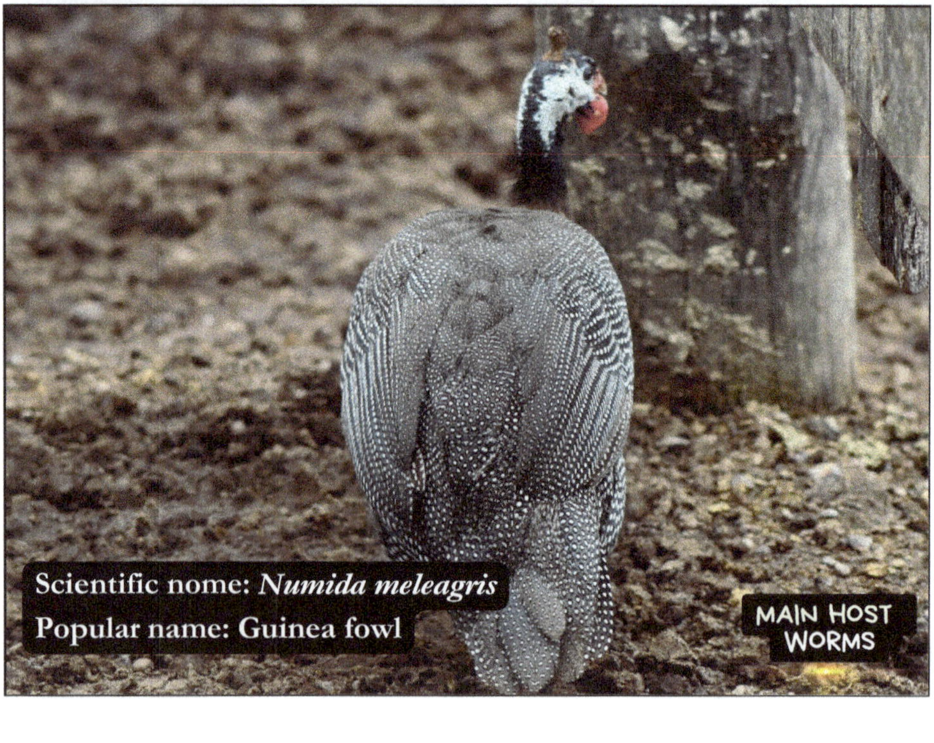
Scientific nome: *Numida meleagris*
Popular name: Guinea fowl
MAIN HOST
WORMS

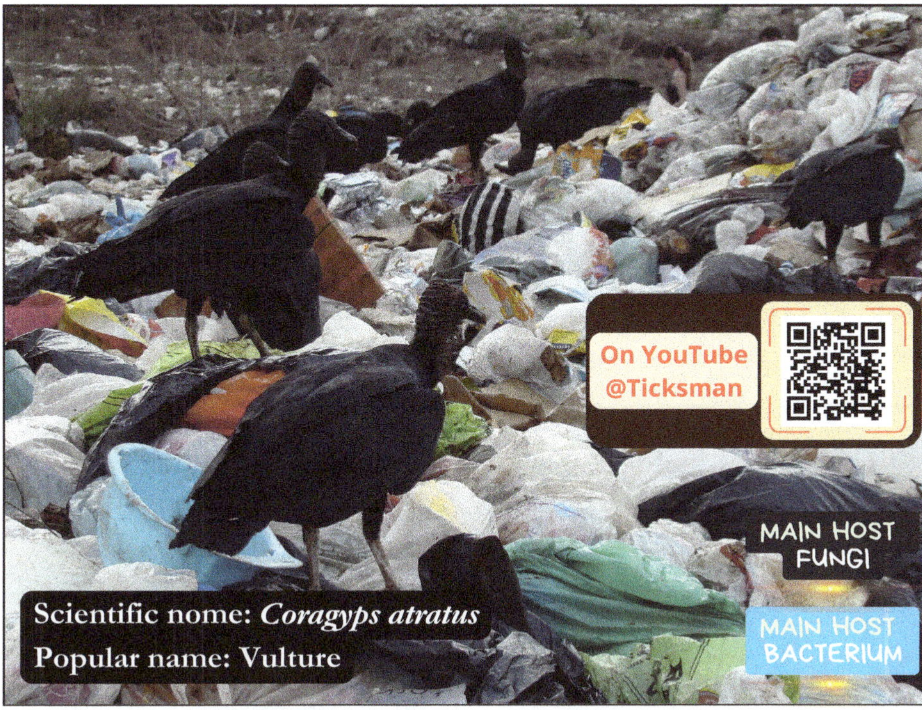
On YouTube
@Ticksman
MAIN HOST
FUNGI
MAIN HOST
BACTERIUM
Scientific nome: *Coragyps atratus*
Popular name: Vulture

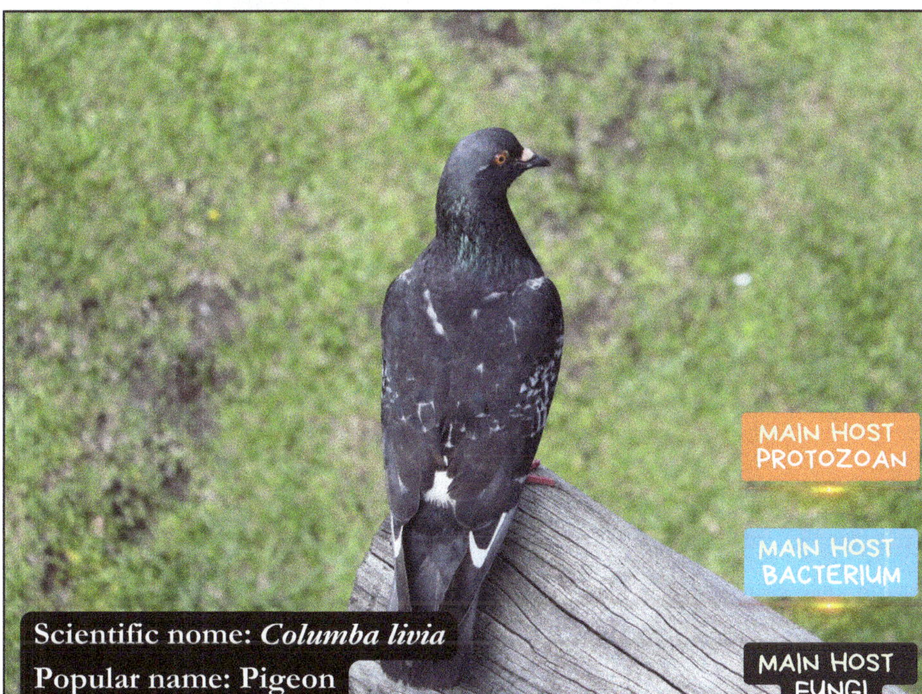
MAIN HOST
PROTOZOAN
MAIN HOST
BACTERIUM
MAIN HOST
FUNGI
Scientific nome: *Columba livia*
Popular name: Pigeon

Domestic & Synanthropic Animals & Their Main Pathogen Groups

This table presents one key disease per domestic or synanthropic animal, based on the pathogen group it most frequently carries or transmits to humans. There are, of course, many other important diseases for each species. You may even disagree with some selections—and that's okay! Our world is diverse, and the prevalence of certain diseases varies greatly depending on the region.

Animal	Main Pathogen Group	Example of Related Disease
Dog	**Protozoa**	*Leishmania infantum* – Canine Leishmaniasis
Cat	**Protozoa**	*Toxoplasma gondii* – Toxoplasmosis
Horse	**Protozoa**	*Babesia caballi, Trypanosoma evansi*
Sheep	**Bacteria**	*Brucella melitensis* – Brucellosis
Vulture	**Bacteria**	*Clostridium* spp., *Salmonella* spp.
Cow	**Bacteria**	*Brucella abortus, Leptospira* spp.
Chicken	**Bacteria**	*Salmonella enterica* – Foodborne Salmonellosis
Duck	**Viruses**	*Avian Influenza* (H5N1)
Guinea fowl	**Worms**	*Ascaridia galli* – Roundworm Infection
Pig	**Worms**	*Taenia solium* – Cysticercosis / Taeniasis
Pigeon	**Fungi**	*Cryptococcus neoformans* – Cryptococcosis

Author's Note:

In my opinion, *Cryptococcus neoformans* – Cryptococcosis is one of the most concerning infections, since we can become infected simply by inhaling its fungal spores. That's why it's so important to be cautious and stay informed about all types of diseases. Prevention starts with awareness!

Diseases Carried by Domestic Animals

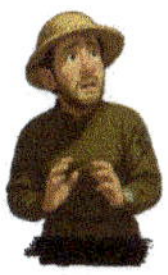

Worms (Helminths) - Ranking: Most Dangerous Helminth Infections to Humans

Discover the five worm-related diseases selected by the author as the most dangerous to humans—each one linked to animals that live closely with us. These animals may carry the parasites without showing any signs, completely unaware of the danger they can silently transmit.

Disease / Pathogen	Main Animal Host	Transmission
**Taenia solium* – Taeniasis / Neurocysticercosis	Pigs	Eating undercooked pork or ingesting feces from infected people.
Echinococcus granulosus – Hydatid Disease	Dogs, Sheep	Ingesting parasite eggs from contaminated food, water, or dog contact.
Trichinella spiralis – Trichinellosis	Pigs	Eating raw or undercooked pork or wild game meat.
Toxocara canis / *T. cati* – Toxocariasis	Dogs, Cats	Ingesting eggs from soil or surfaces contaminated with animal feces.
Ancylostoma caninum / *A. braziliense* – Hookworm Infection	Dogs, Cats	Skin contact with contaminated soil or sand.

*See example below

Disease: Taeniasis / Neurocysticercosis (*Taenia solium*)

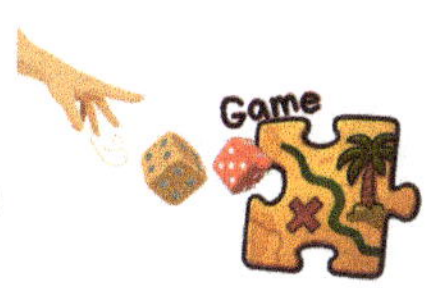

Transmission / Vectors

Humans get taeniasis by eating undercooked pork with larvae (cysticerci).

Neurocysticercosis happens when a person accidentally swallows eggs from human feces (poor hygiene or contaminated food/water).

Signs and Symptoms

Taeniasis: Often no symptoms, or mild stomach discomfort.

Neurocysticercosis: Headaches, seizures, confusion, and neurological problems.

Diagnosis / Tests

Stool tests for eggs or segments.

CT scans or MRIs to detect cysts in the brain for neurocysticercosis.

Prevention / Prophylaxis

Wash hands often, cook pork thoroughly, improve sanitation, and treat infected individuals to stop egg spreading.

Treatment

Taeniasis: Antiparasitic drugs.

Neurocysticercosis: If neurocysticercosis is suspected, go to the hospital immediately. A doctor will confirm the diagnosis and begin the correct treatment. Do not self-medicate.

Geographic Distribution

Found in Latin America, Sub-Saharan Africa, Asia, and areas with poor sanitation and free-range pig farming.

Attention: When planning a trip, be aware of regional and local diseases.

Major Helminthic Infections and Their Key Characteristics

This table presents four of the most important parasitic worm infections transmitted by animals or contaminated environments. It summarizes how each disease is acquired, its main symptoms, how it's diagnosed, and the most effective prevention methods. Always consult a healthcare professional for diagnosis and treatment—worms can be sneaky, but with the right knowledge, we can outsmart them!

Characteristics	**Hydatid Disease** (*Echinococcus granulosus*)	**Trichinellosis** (*Trichinella spiralis*)	**Toxocariasis** (*Toxocara canis / T. cati*)	**Hookworm Infection** (*Ancylostoma* spp.)
Transmission / Vectors	Ingestion of parasite eggs via contaminated food, water, or contact with infected dog feces	Eating undercooked pork or wild game meat containing larvae	Ingestion of eggs from soil or surfaces contaminated with pet feces	Skin contact with soil contaminated with larvae (walking barefoot)
Signs and Symptoms	Often asymptomatic; can cause cysts in liver, lungs, brain—pain, nausea, organ dysfunction	Fever, muscle pain, swelling around eyes, diarrhea, weakness	Cough, fever, abdominal pain, vision loss (ocular larva migrans)	Itchy rash ("creeping eruption"), abdominal pain, anemia
Diagnosis / Tests	Ultrasound, CT/MRI scans, serology (ELISA)	Blood tests, muscle biopsy, serology	Blood tests (ELISA), eye exam (for ocular form)	Stool exam, blood test for anemia
Prevention / Prophylaxis	Wash hands, deworm dogs, avoid consuming unwashed vegetables or contaminated food	Cook meat thoroughly, avoid raw or undercooked pork/game	Deworm pets, clean up pet feces, teach kids proper hygiene	Wear shoes outdoors, improve sanitation, avoid walking barefoot
Treatment	Exists; medical and sometimes surgical; always under medical supervision	Exists; early treatment important; see a doctor if exposed	Exists; treatment depends on severity and location of larvae	Exists; doctor will prescribe treatment; avoid self-medication
Geographic Distribution	Endemic in areas with sheep farming and dogs: Mediterranean, South America, Central Asia	Worldwide, especially in regions where raw/undercooked meat is consumed	Worldwide; more common in areas with stray dogs and poor sanitation	Tropical and subtropical areas; common in Latin America, Africa, Southeast Asia

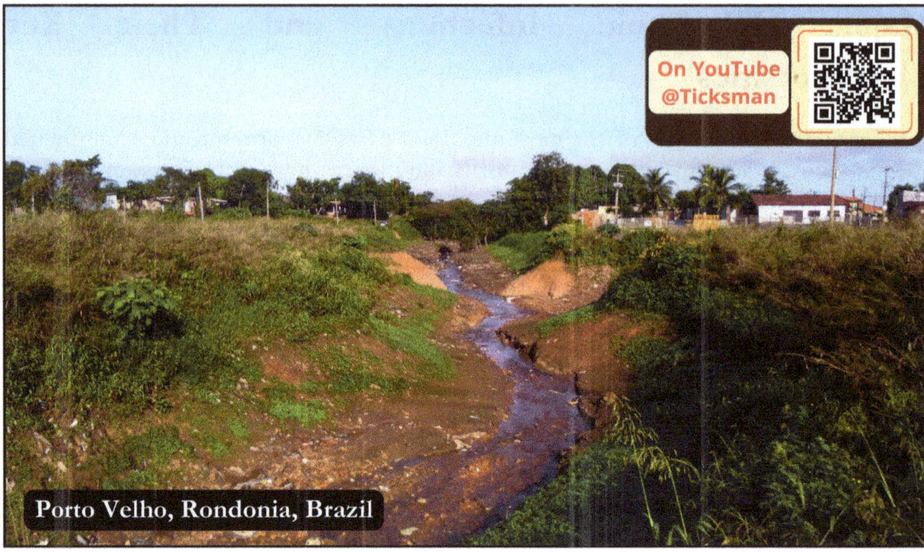

Porto Velho, Rondonia, Brazil

In urban areas like this one, where streams run between houses, human waste—such as feces and urine—is often dumped directly into the water. As a result, people can become infected with various diseases, including parasitic worm eggs.

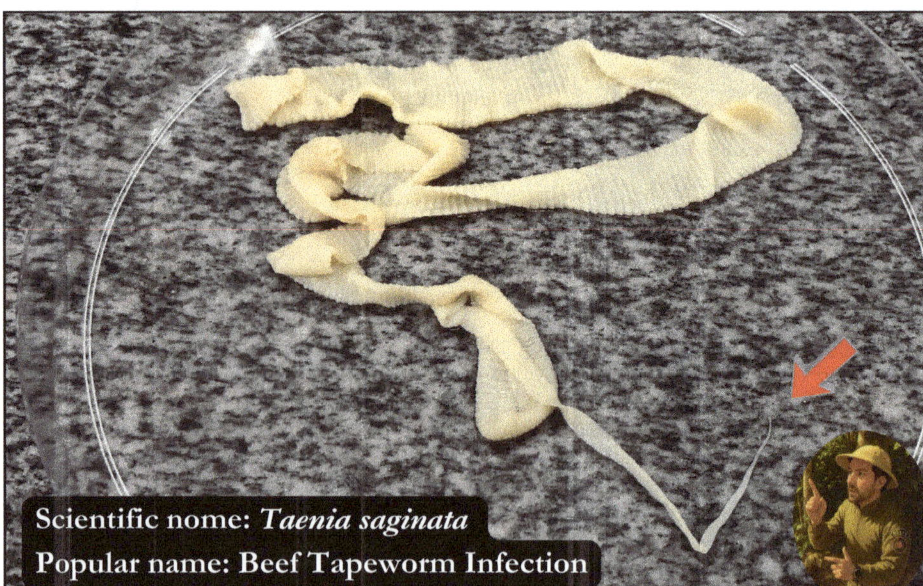
Scientific nome: *Taenia saginata*
Popular name: Beef Tapeworm Infection

In this image, you can see an adult tapeworm with its body segments (called proglottids) and the narrow end known as the scolex, which attaches to the wall of the human small intestine. Each proglottid can produce up to 100,000 eggs that are released in human feces. This species is less dangerous than the pork tapeworm (*Taenia solium*), which can cause neurocysticercosis.

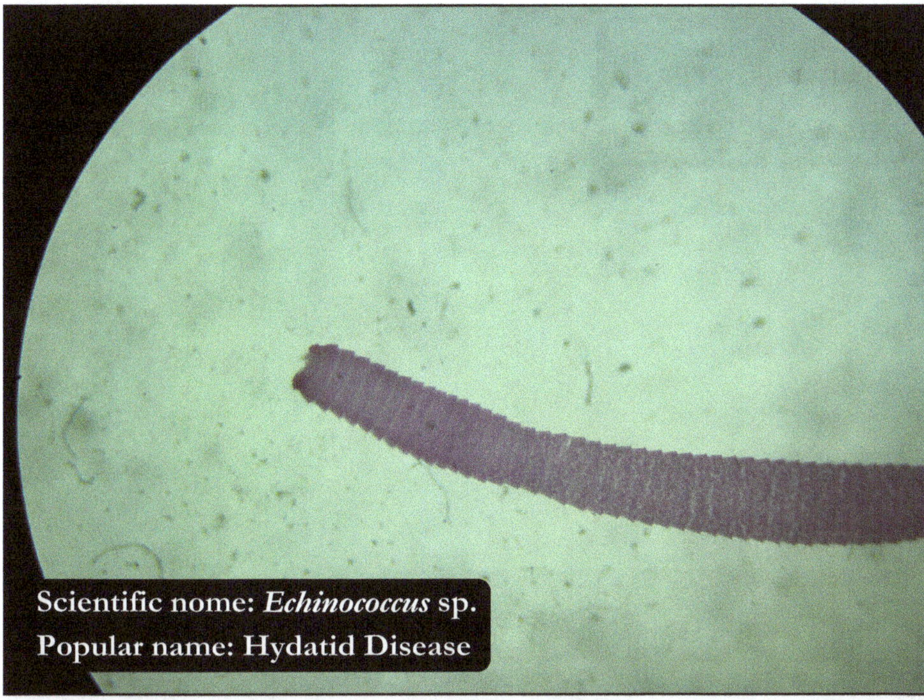

Scientific nome: *Echinococcus* sp.
Popular name: Hydatid Disease

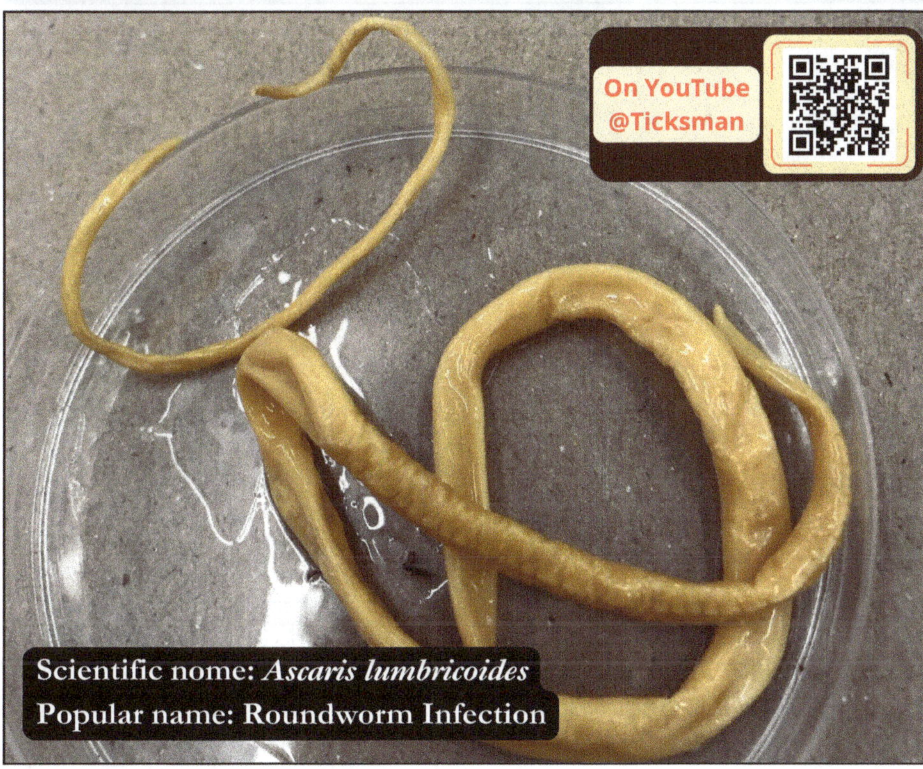

Scientific nome: *Ascaris lumbricoides*
Popular name: Roundworm Infection

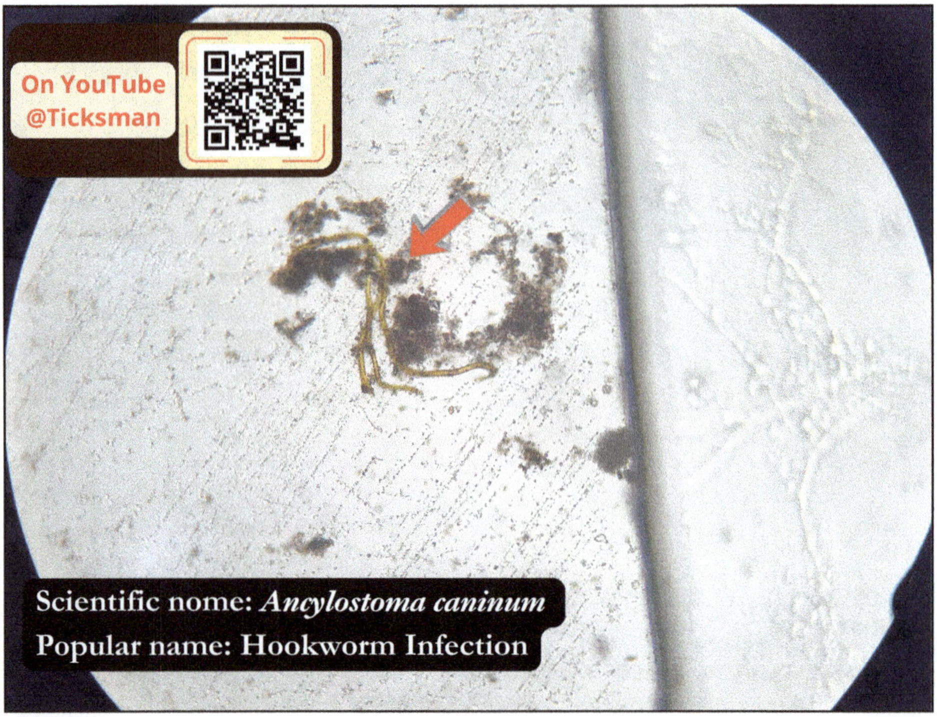

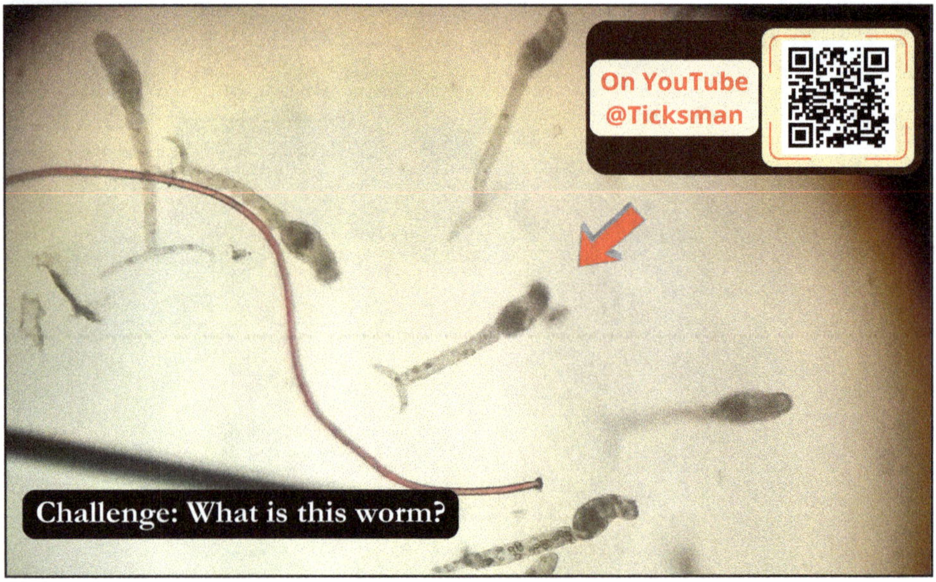

Parasite Challenge: This strange-looking worm is in its second stage after hatching from an egg. Native to Africa, it has already spread to parts of the Americas and Asia. With its distinctive forked tail, it swims freely and can penetrate human skin—especially between 10 a.m. and 2 p.m.—causing intense itching. Can you guess what it is?

General Prevention Tips for Helminth Infections

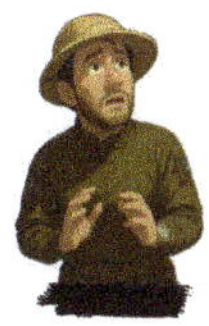
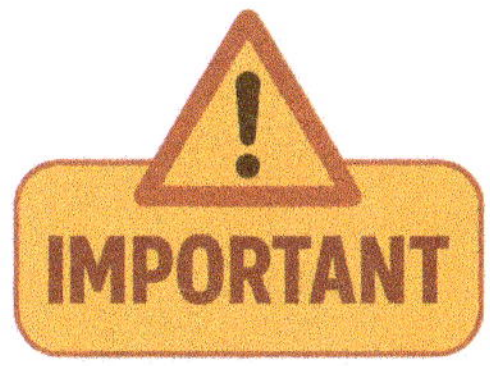

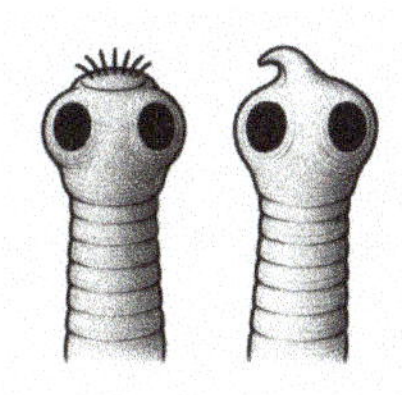

I. Cook Meat Thoroughly

- Always cook pork, beef, and poultry to safe internal temperatures.
- Avoid raw or undercooked sausages, bacon, and game meats.

II. Wash Hands Regularly

- Especially after handling pets, soil, or cleaning litter boxes.
- Use soap and water—especially before meals or cooking.

III. Deworm Pets Routinely

- Consult veterinarians for scheduled antiparasitic treatments for dogs and cats.
- Clean pet bedding and waste areas frequently.

IV. Avoid Walking Barefoot in Soil

- Especially in areas where dogs or cats roam.
- Use sandals or closed shoes in parks, sandboxes, gardens.

V. Wash Fruits and Vegetables Thoroughly

- Especially those grown close to the ground or in manure-fertilized soil.

VI. Control Rodents and Wild Animal Exposure

- Keep food and waste secured to avoid contamination by pigs, foxes, rats, or other carriers.

VII. Educate Children

- Teach kids not to put soil, fingers, or objects in their mouths when playing outside.

Now that we understand how each of these worm-related diseases can be transmitted and acquired, the next question is: what can we do at home to ensure no one gets sick from them? The answer starts with awareness and action.

If you have a pet, you already know the importance of regular visits to the veterinarian and keeping their vaccination and deworming schedule up to date. But there's more you can do!

Maintain a clean home and yard, cook your food thoroughly—especially meat—and always wash your hands after handling soil, animals, or raw food.

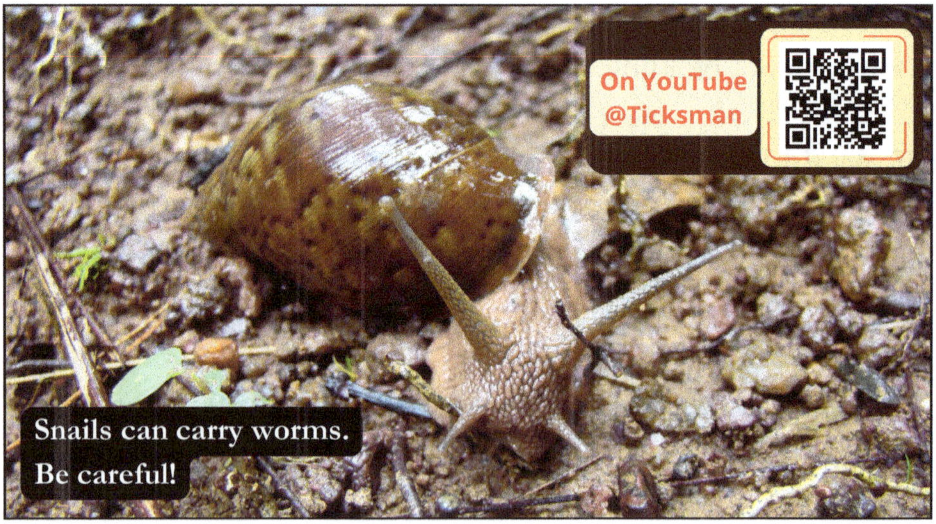

This snail is slowly making its way across the forest floor in the Amazon. But could it be carrying a hidden parasite inside?

Teach children to respect nature but avoid putting unwashed objects in their mouths. Simple habits like wearing shoes outside, washing fruits and vegetables, and not letting pets sleep in beds can greatly reduce the risk of infection.

Your home can become a fortress against parasitic worms—armed with knowledge, hygiene, and love for both people and pets. Prevention is not just a choice; it's a superpower.

Every $1 invested in prevention saves around $4 in treatment and lost productivity. Prevention is not just smart — it's cost-effective. Make it a daily habit!

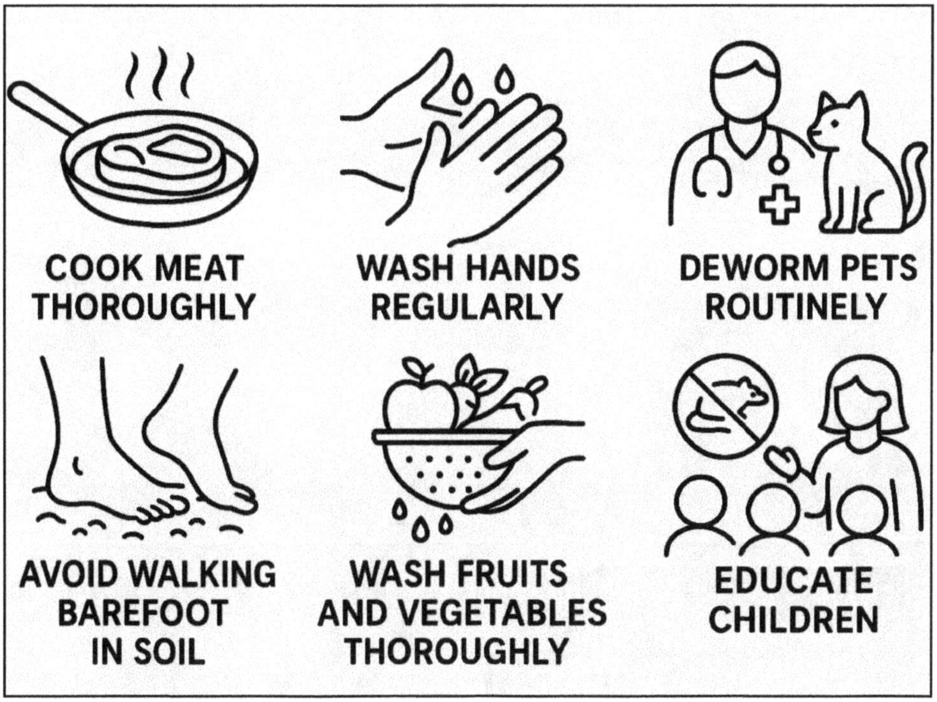

Following these simple daily actions can greatly reduce the risk of parasitic infections. Washing your hands before meals, properly cooking meat and fish, drinking safe water, and keeping your living spaces clean are powerful habits. These actions may seem small, but they make a big difference—protecting not only your own health but also your family, friends, and community. The more people who follow these steps, the fewer parasites we allow to spread. Prevention starts at home, every single day!

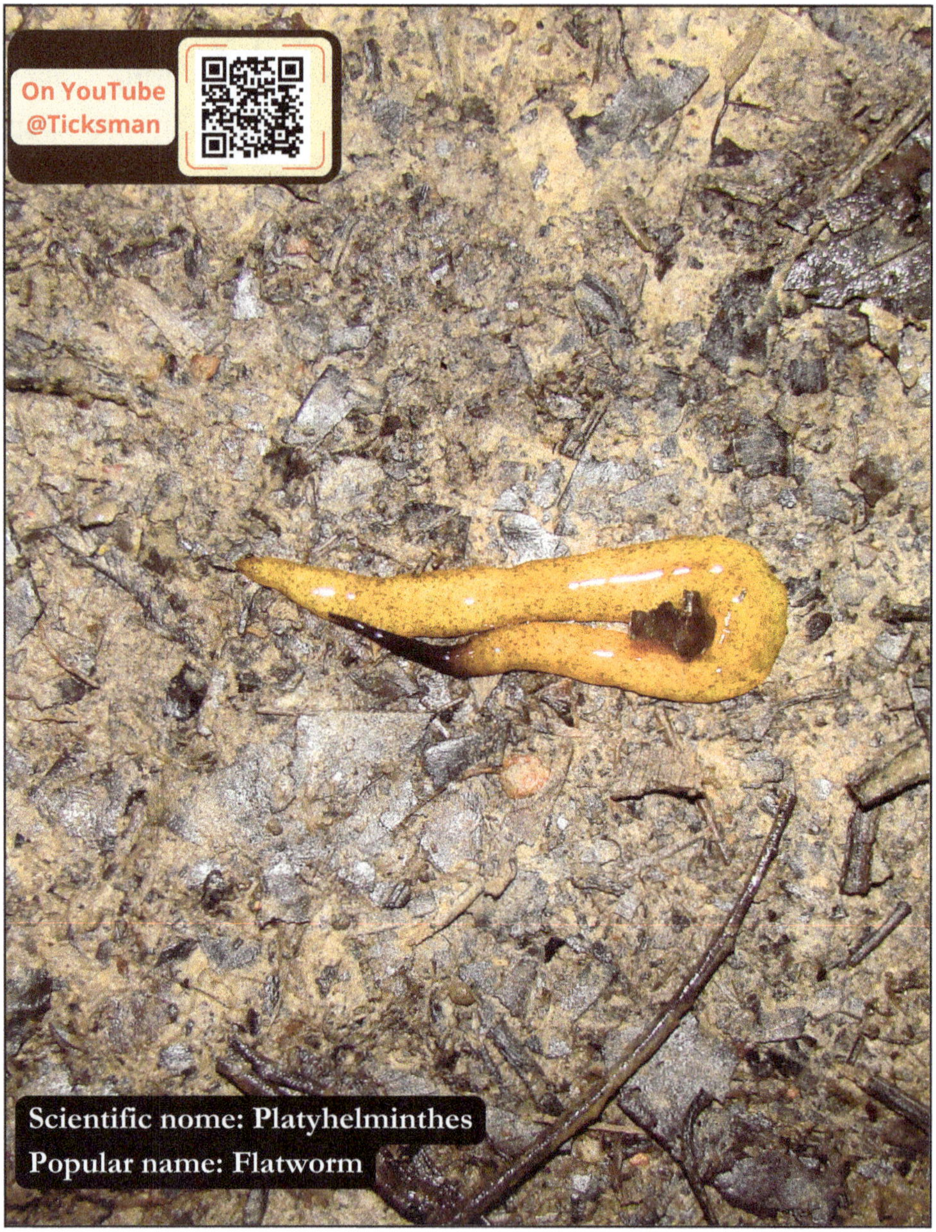

Did you know? Some flatworms are free-living creatures that crawl around at night and feed mainly on earthworms! While they pose no danger to humans, certain invasive species are causing ecological imbalances in parts of the world where they've been introduced—mainly because they have no natural predators in those regions. Despite their slug-like appearance, they are not mollusks and have no visible eyes—a curious detail that sets them apart!

Diseases Carried by Domestic Animals

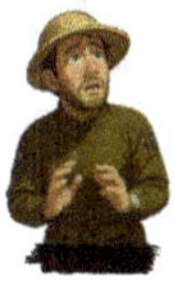

Ranking: Most Dangerous Protozoan Diseases to Humans

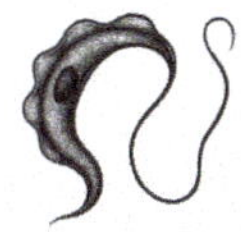

Here are five of the most important protozoan diseases linked to domestic animals. Notice: Malaria, the deadliest protozoan infection in humans, isn't listed here—because it requires an infected person, not a domestic animal, for the mosquito to transmit it.

Disease / Pathogen	Main Animal Host/Reservoir	Transmission
Trypanosoma cruzi – Chagas Disease	Opossums, armadillos, dogs	Feces of assassin bugs, blood transfusion, organ transplant, congenital.
**Toxoplasma gondii* – Toxoplasmosis	Cats	Ingestion of oocysts from cat feces, soil, or undercooked meat.
Leishmania infantum – Leishmaniasis	Dogs, wild canids	Bite of infected sandflies.
Cryptosporidium parvum – Cryptosporidiosis	Cattle, goats	Ingestion of oocysts through contaminated water or food.
Giardia duodenalis – Giardiasis	Dogs, cats, livestock	Fecal-oral route via contaminated water, food, or direct contact.

*See example below

Author's Note:

Chagas disease is increasingly gaining global attention, with over 300,000 cases reported in the United States, 80,000 in Europe, and 20,000 in Asia—regions where the triatomine "Assassin bug" vector is not naturally endemic. In these areas, transmission has occurred primarily due to the lack of mandatory screening for Chagas disease in blood and organ donors. As large numbers of migrants from South America—where the disease is endemic—arrive, undetected chronic infections are being introduced.

▲ Chronic Chagas disease has no cure, which makes awareness and prevention critical. Stay informed and help spread this important message.

Disease: Toxoplasmosis - (*Toxoplasma gondii*)

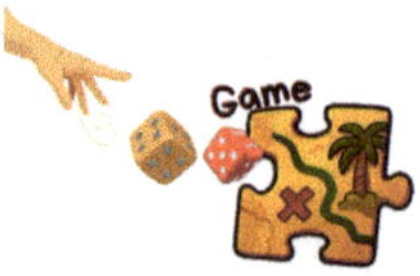

Transmission / Vectors

Primarily transmitted through ingestion of oocysts from cat feces, contaminated soil, or undercooked meat (especially pork or lamb).

Also possible through mother-to-baby transmission (congenital) and organ transplants.

Signs and Symptoms

Often asymptomatic in healthy people.

When symptoms occur: mild fever, swollen lymph nodes, fatigue.

In pregnant women: may cause miscarriage or birth defects.

In immunocompromised people: risk of encephalitis and severe complications.

Diagnosis / Tests

Blood tests to detect antibodies (IgG, IgM).

Imaging (MRI/CT) in severe or neurological cases.

Amniotic fluid PCR for fetal infection.

Prevention / Prophylaxis

Avoid contact with cat litter and raw meat.

Wash fruits/vegetables, cook meat thoroughly.

Wear gloves while gardening.

Pregnant women should avoid handling raw meat or cat litter.

Protozoan Diseases and Their Impact on Human Health

Protozoa are single-celled organisms capable of causing significant illness in humans. This table presents four key protozoan infections, summarizing how they spread, their symptoms, and how to prevent them. Some are spread by insect bites, others through contaminated water—understanding these tiny invaders helps us protect ourselves and our families.

Characteristics	Chagas Disease	Leishmaniasis	Cryptosporidiosis	Giardiasis
Transmission / Vectors	Feces of infected kissing bugs (assassin bugs)	Bite of infected sandflies	Contaminated water, fecal-oral	Contaminated water, fecal-oral
Signs and Symptoms	Fever, swelling (Romana's sign), fatigue, possible chronic heart/ digestive damage	Skin sores (cutaneous) or fever, weight loss, organ enlargement (visceral)	Watery diarrhea, nausea, stomach cramps	Diarrhea, gas, bloating, cramps
Diagnosis / Tests	Blood test, PCR, serology	Microscopy, PCR, biopsy	Stool test, antigen detection	Stool test, antigen detection
Prevention / Prophylaxis	Vector control, housing improvements, hygiene	Avoid sandfly bites, protect pets, vector control	Drink treated water, good sanitation	Boil/filter water, hygiene
Treatment	Requires medical treatment—see a doctor	Requires medical treatment—see a doctor	Supportive care, medical treatment needed	Supportive care, medical treatment needed
Geographic Distribution	Endemic in Latin America; also cases in U.S., Europe	Latin America, Mediterranean, Middle East, Asia	Worldwide, especially in low-sanitation areas	Worldwide, especially in children

Treatment

- Most healthy individuals don't need treatment.
- If toxoplasmosis is suspected—especially in pregnant individuals or those with weakened immune systems—it is crucial to seek medical attention immediately. Be sure to inform the doctor if you've had contact with raw or undercooked meat, unwashed fruits or vegetables, unpasteurized milk, or cat feces.

The physician will order specific tests and, once the diagnosis is confirmed, will prescribe the appropriate treatment based on the patient's condition. Never self-medicate—only a healthcare professional can determine the correct course of action.

Geographic Distribution

- Worldwide—higher prevalence in warm, humid climates and regions with lower food safety.

Very common in Latin America, Africa, and parts of Europe.

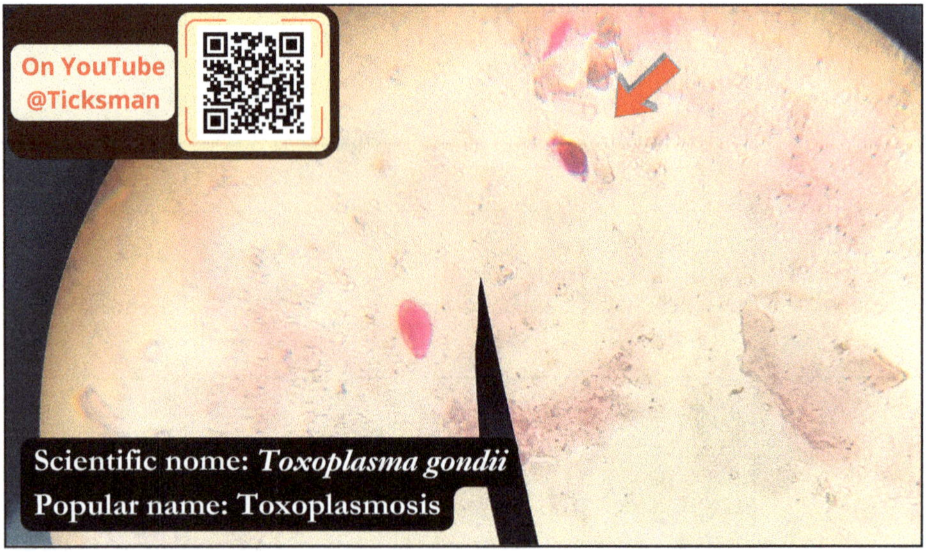

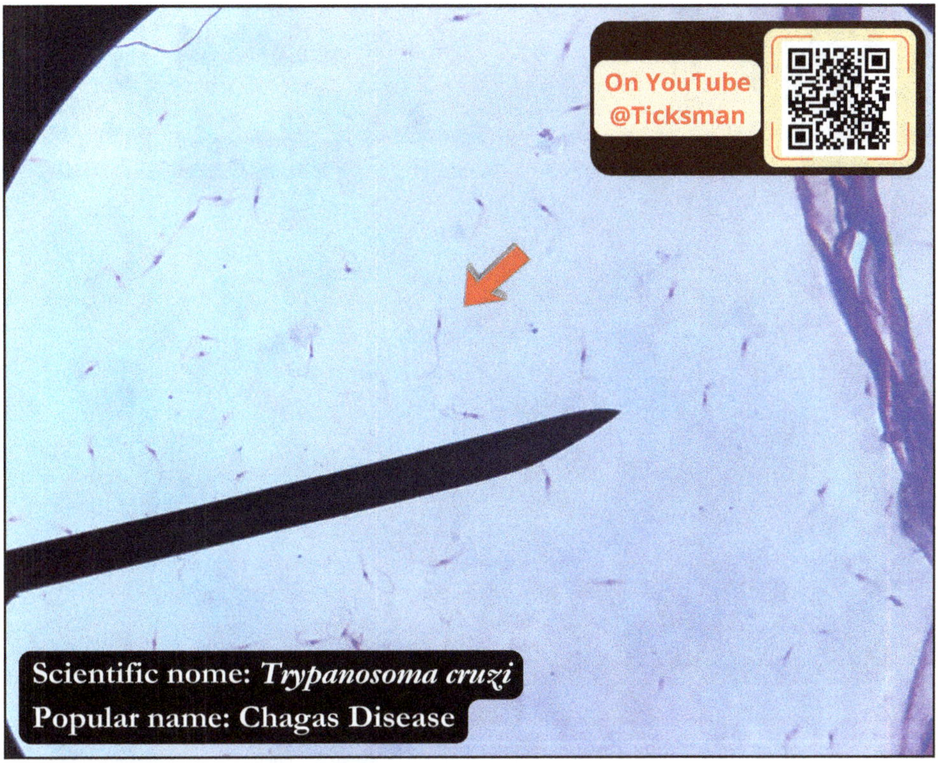
On YouTube
@Ticksman
Scientific nome: *Trypanosoma cruzi*
Popular name: Chagas Disease

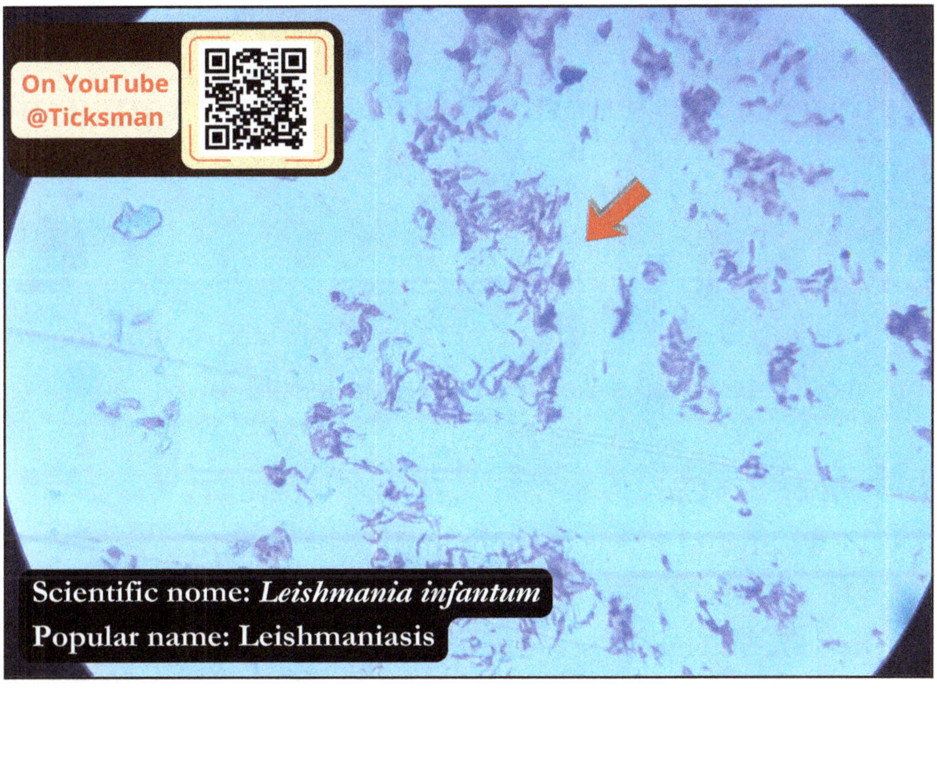
On YouTube
@Ticksman
Scientific nome: *Leishmania infantum*
Popular name: Leishmaniasis

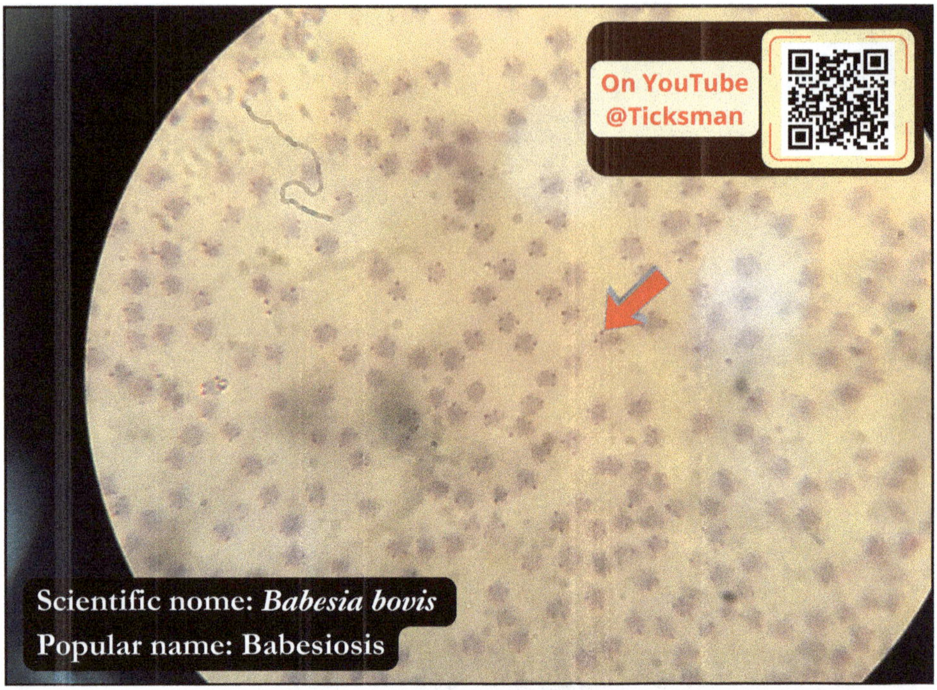

In this image under 40x magnification, mammalian cells are shown infected with the protozoan *Babesia*. The small red dots inside the cells are the parasites.

General Prevention Tips for Protozoan Infections

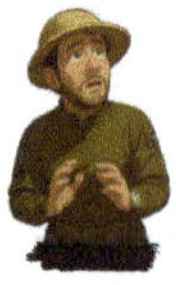

I. Avoid Contact with Infected Insects

- Use repellents, mosquito nets, and protective clothing to avoid bites from sandflies, ticks, and kissing bugs.

II. Proper Pet Care

- Deworm and vaccinate dogs and cats regularly.
- Do not allow pets to roam freely in areas where they can become infected.

III. Handle Cat Litter Safely

- Pregnant women should avoid cleaning litter boxes or wear gloves and wash hands thoroughly.

IV. Cook Meat Thoroughly

- Avoid undercooked lamb, pork, and beef, especially to prevent toxoplasmosis and giardiasis.

V. Drink Clean, Safe Water

- Use filtered or boiled water, especially in rural or forested ar

VI. Wash Hands Frequently

- Especially after handling animals, working in the garden, or preparing raw meat.

VII. Avoid Blood Exposure

- Be cautious with blood transfusions and organ transplants, particularly in endemic areas for Chagas disease or babesiosis.

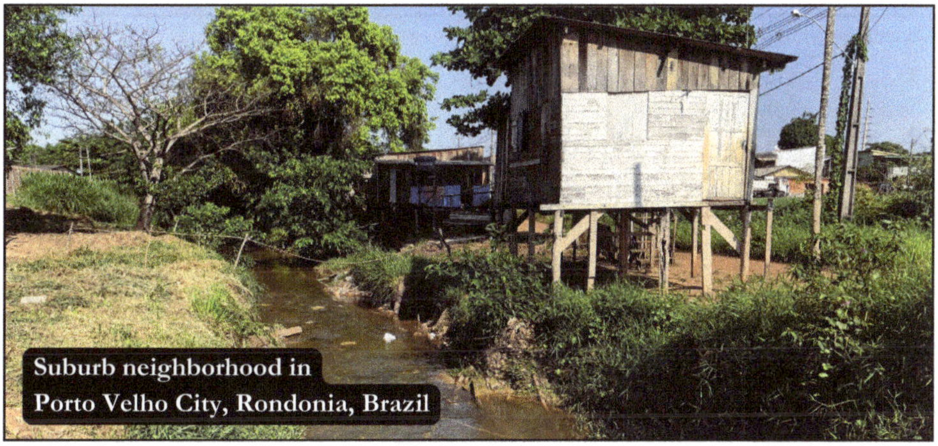
Suburb neighborhood in
Porto Velho City, Rondonia, Brazil

This photo shows a stilt house in an Amazonian town. The lack of basic sanitation is critical and contributes to the spread of parasitic diseases. Be careful: always treat your water and never dump human waste or garbage into rivers and streams.

Bacteria – Ranking: Top 5 Most Significant Human Infections

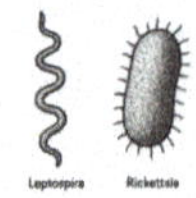

The table below presents five major bacterial diseases transmitted by vectors—such as insects, arachnids, or through direct contact with contaminated surfaces or fluids. If not diagnosed and treated promptly by a doctor, these infections can lead to hospitalization, severe complications, or even death.

Disease / Pathogen	Main Animal Host/Reservoir	Transmission
**Leptospira* spp. – Leptospirosis	Dogs, cattle, pigs, rodents	Contact with urine of infected animals; often through contaminated water or soil.
**Rickettsia rickettsii* – RMSF	Dogs, wild mammals (via ticks)	Bite of infected ticks, especially *Amblyomma* spp. and *Dermacentor* spp.
Brucella spp. – Brucellosis	Cattle, pigs, sheep, goats	Contact with infected fluids, raw dairy products, or undercooked meat.
Salmonella spp. – Salmonellosis	Poultry, reptiles, mammals	Eating contaminated eggs, meat, or contact with infected animals.
Campylobacter jejuni – Campylobacteriosis	Chickens, cattle	Ingestion of undercooked poultry or contaminated water/milk.

*See example below

Disease: Leptospirosis - (*Leptospira* spp.)

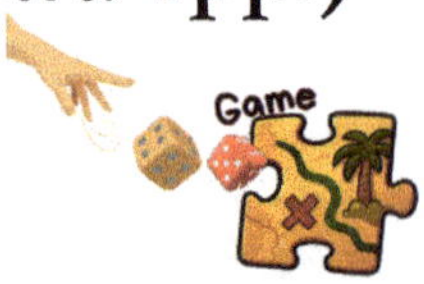

Transmission / Vectors

Transmitted through direct contact with urine of infected animals (especially rodents, dogs, pigs, cattle), or indirectly through contaminated water, soil, or mud.

Common in floodwaters and tropical environments.

Disease: Leptospirosis - (*Leptospira* spp.)

Transmission / Vectors

Transmitted through direct contact with urine of infected animals (especially rodents, dogs, pigs, cattle), or indirectly through contaminated water, soil, or mud.

Common in floodwaters and tropical environments.

Signs and Symptoms

Sudden fever, headache, muscle pain (especially calves), chills, vomiting, red eyes.

Severe cases may lead to kidney or liver failure, meningitis, hemorrhages, or Weil's disease.

Diagnosis / Tests

Blood or urine tests (PCR, MAT test).

May require repeated tests due to variation in bacterial levels.

Prevention / Prophylaxis

Avoid contact with stagnant or flood water.

Wear protective gear during outdoor or farm work.

Boil or treat drinking water in at-risk areas.

Control rodent populations.

Treatment

Early antibiotic treatment: A doctor will confirm the diagnosis and begin the correct treatment. Do not self-medicate.

Hospital care for severe cases with organ complications.

Geographic Distribution

Found worldwide, especially in tropical and subtropical areas, rural or urban slums, and places prone to flooding.

Disease: Rocky Mountain Spotted Fever (RMSF) - (*Rickettsia rickettsii*)

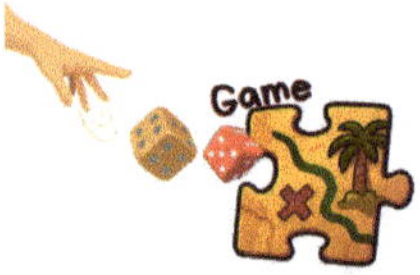

Also known as RMSF in the U.S.

Known as Brazilian Spotted Fever (Febre Maculosa Brasileira) in Brazil

Transmission / Vectors

Transmitted by the bite of infected ticks:

U.S.: *Dermacentor variabilis* (American dog tick) and *Dermacentor andersoni*

Brazil: *Amblyomma sculptum* and *Amblyomma aureolatum* (commonly found on horses and dogs)

Signs and Symptoms

High fever, severe headache, muscle pain, nausea, and vomiting.

Rash appears 2–5 days after fever begins (may start on wrists/ankles).

Without treatment, can lead to organ failure and death.

Diagnosis / Tests

Blood test with PCR or indirect immunofluorescence (IFA).

! Early diagnosis is challenging but crucial — treatment should begin based on symptoms and risk.

Prevention / Prophylaxis

🧴 Use tick repellents (DEET), wear protective clothing.

🔍 Perform full body tick checks after walking in forests or tall grass.

🐕 Keep pets tick-free and out of tick-infested areas.

🌳 In rural Brazil, avoid grassy areas with free-roaming animals.

Treatment

A doctor will confirm the diagnosis and begin the correct treatment. Do not self-medicate.

⏱ Treatment should begin immediately if RMSF is suspected, even before test results.

Geographic Distribution

● Found in North, Central, and South America.

▲ High-risk regions:

U.S.: United States: Primarily in the southeastern and south-central states; however, cases have been reported throughout the contiguous U.S.

Brazil: Predominantly in the Southeast region, including São Paulo, Minas Gerais, Espírito Santo, and Rio de Janeiro. Notably, cases have also been identified in southern states such as Santa Catarina and Rio Grande do Sul.

Other countries: Documented in Mexico, Panama, Costa Rica, Colombia, and Argentina.

Common Zoonotic Bacterial Infections

This table highlights three major bacterial diseases transmitted through food or direct contact with animals. Proper food handling, personal hygiene, and avoiding raw animal products are key strategies for prevention. These infections may start mild but can become severe if left untreated.

Characteristics	Brucellosis	Salmonellosis	Campylobacteriosis
Transmission / Vectors	Contact with infected animal fluids, raw milk/ meat	Fecal-oral from contaminated food (eggs, poultry)	Ingestion of undercooked chicken or unpasteurized milk
Signs and Symptoms	Fever, joint pain, fatigue, night sweats	Diarrhea, abdominal cramps, vomiting	Diarrhea, abdominal pain, fever
Diagnosis / Tests	Blood test, serology, culture	Stool culture, PCR	Stool culture, PCR
Prevention / Prophylaxis	Avoid raw dairy/ meat, wear gloves on farms	Cook food thoroughly, kitchen hygiene	Safe food handling, hygiene practices
Treatment	Requires medical treatment—see a doctor	Supportive care or antibiotics—doctor required	Supportive care or antibiotics—doctor required
Geographic Distribution	Global, more common in rural/ farming areas	Worldwide	Worldwide

General Prevention Tips for Bacterial Zoonoses

I. Wash Hands Frequently

- Especially after handling animals, cleaning litter boxes, or working outdoors.
- Use soap and running water for at least 20 seconds.

II. Cook Food Properly

- Ensure meat, eggs, and dairy products are cooked to safe temperatures.
- Avoid raw milk and undercooked pork or poultry.

III. Avoid Contact with Animal Urine

- Use protective gear when working in farms or flood-affected areas.
- Don't swim in or drink from stagnant or suspicious water sources.

IV. Control Ticks and Fleas

- Keep pets on a tick prevention schedule.
- Maintain clean surroundings and inspect animals regularly.

V. Vaccinate Your Pets

- Dogs and livestock should be vaccinated against Leptospira and Brucella when recommended.

VI. Handle Animal Bites Promptly

- Wash wounds with soap and water and seek medical attention if bitten by a pet or stray animal.

VII. Practice Safe Food Handling

- Keep raw meat separate, refrigerate perishables, and clean surfaces and utensils thoroughly.

Remember: Bacterial infections often begin with the invisible—microscopic exposure through bites, scratches, food, or water.

But with the right hygiene, veterinary care, and awareness, we can keep these invisible invaders from causing real danger.

Viruses – Ranking: Top 5 Most Significant Viral Infections

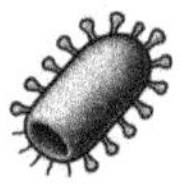

The table below highlights five major viruses transmitted to humans through animals. Pay special attention to Hantavirus, which is featured in the next section of our Parasite Dice Game.

Disease / Pathogen	Main Animal Host/Reservoir	Transmission
Rabies virus – Rabies	Dogs, cats, bats	Bite from infected animals; saliva exposure.
**Hantavirus* – Hantavirus Pulmonary Syndrome (HPS)	Rodents	Inhalation of aerosolized urine or feces from infected rodents.
Influenza A viruses – Avian & Swine Flu	Poultry, pigs	Contact with infected animals or their secretions.
Newcastle disease virus – Newcastle Disease	Chickens, other birds	Handling infected birds or contact with their droppings or secretions.
Feline leukemia virus (FeLV) – Feline Leukemia	Cats	Through saliva, nasal secretions, grooming, and shared food/water bowls.

*See example below

Major Viral Diseases Related to Animals

This table summarizes key viral infections transmitted by animals or through close contact. While some like FeLV affect only animals, others such as rabies and flu pose significant risks to humans. Vaccination, early diagnosis, and avoiding exposure to potentially infected animals remain the best protective strategies.

Characteristics	Rabies	Avian & Swine Flu	Newcastle Disease	Feline Leukemia (FeLV)
Transmission / Vectors	Saliva from bites of infected animals (dogs, bats)	Contact with infected birds/ pigs or secretions	Contact with infected birds or surfaces	Saliva, nasal secretions between cats
Signs and Symptoms	Confusion, fever, paralysis, death	Fever, cough, sore throat, fatigue	Mild conjunctivitis (in humans)	Weakness, weight loss, infections, anemia
Diagnosis / Tests	Clinical signs, post-mortem brain test	Nasal swab PCR, serology	Virus isolation or antibody testing	Blood test (ELISA or IFA)
Prevention / Prophylaxis	Rabies vaccination, avoid stray animals	Vaccination (for animals), hygiene	Biosecurity in poultry farms	FeLV vaccination, testing cats regularly
Treatment	No cure after symptoms—emergency care needed	Supportive care only—see a doctor	No specific treatment—supportive care	No cure, supportive care—see a vet
Geographic Distribution	Worldwide (especially Asia, Africa)	Global outbreaks (varies by strain)	Worldwide (in poultry)	Worldwide (domestic cats)

Disease: Hantavirus Pulmonary Syndrome (HPS) - (*Hantavirus*)

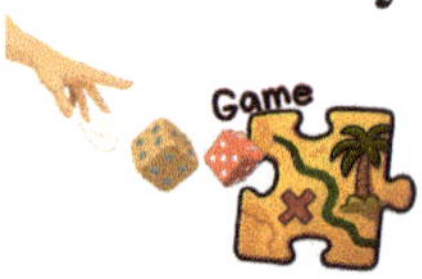

Transmission / Vectors

Transmitted by inhalation of aerosolized particles from urine, droppings, or saliva of infected wild rodents (especially deer mice).

Not transmitted from person to person in most cases.

Signs and Symptoms

Early: Fever, muscle aches (especially in thighs and back), fatigue, headache, dizziness.

Later: Sudden shortness of breath, fluid in lungs, low blood pressure — can be life-threatening.

Diagnosis / Tests

Blood tests for hantavirus antibodies (IgM, IgG) or PCR.

Chest X-ray to detect pulmonary edema (fluid in lungs).

Prevention / Prophylaxis

Avoid sweeping rodent-infested areas.

Disinfect urine/droppings with bleach before cleaning.

Seal entry points to prevent rodent access in homes or storage areas.

Wear gloves and masks during cleanup.

Treatment

🏥 No specific antiviral treatment — supportive care is essential. A doctor will confirm the diagnosis and begin the correct treatment. Do not self-medicate.

🫁 Hospitalization with oxygen therapy or intensive care may be needed.

Geographic Distribution

🌍 Found in the Americas, especially the U.S., Argentina, Chile, and Brazil.

Linked to rural areas, cabins, and grain storage facilities.

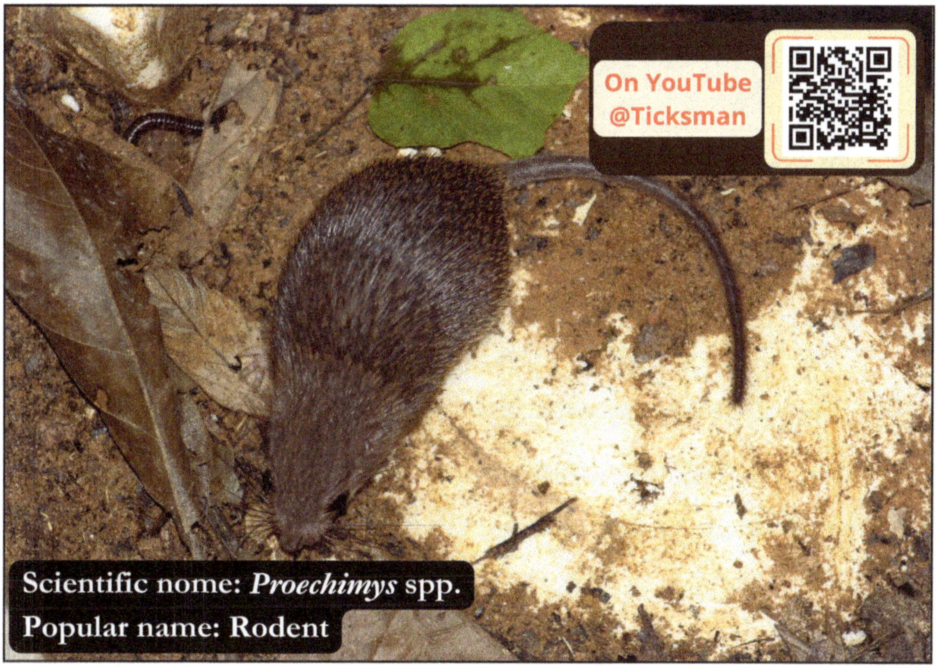
On YouTube
@Ticksman
Scientific nome: *Proechimys* spp.
Popular name: Rodent

Rodents of the genus *Proechimys* spp., like the one shown in this photo taken in the Amazon rainforest, serve as reservoirs for various pathogens. They can remain asymptomatic for long periods, silently maintaining the transmission cycle in nature. However, they too can become sick and die, especially when infected by aggressive viral agents. This highlights the delicate balance between wildlife and disease ecology in tropical environments.

General Prevention Tips for Viral Zoonoses

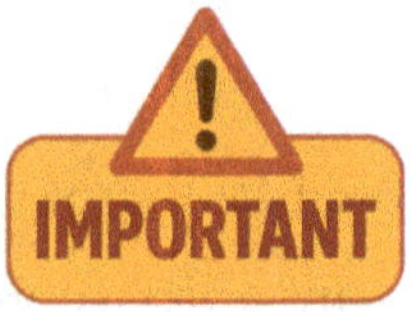

I. Vaccinate Pets Regularly

- Keep your dog's rabies and distemper vaccines updated.
- Ensure cats are protected against FeLV and FIV.

II. Avoid Contact with Stray or Wild Animals

- Especially bats, raccoons, and stray dogs or cats.
- Report animals acting strangely to local health authorities.

III. Use Personal Protection in Farms

- Wear gloves, masks, and boots when handling poultry or pigs.
- Wash hands thoroughly after animal contact.

IV. Control Rodent Populations

- Keep homes clean and seal food to avoid attracting rodents.
- Clean rodent droppings with gloves and masks—never sweep or vacuum dried droppings.

V. Practice Good Hygiene with Pets

- Don't let pets lick your face or wounds.
- Attention: Take your pets to the vet periodically.
- Clean litter boxes and cages frequently (especially for indoor cats).

VI. Stay Informed About Outbreaks

- Monitor local health bulletins for viral outbreaks in animals or humans.
- Avoid traveling to outbreak zones when possible.

Viral diseases remind us that even invisible threats can have powerful consequences—but with vaccines, hygiene, and awareness, we can build strong barriers against them.

Prevention is protection!

Fungi – Ranking: Top 5 Most Significant Human Mycoses

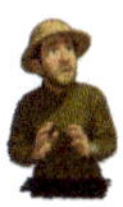

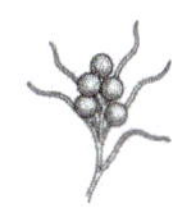

Fungal diseases are often overlooked, but they are just as important—and sometimes just as deadly—as any other group presented in this book. The table below highlights five of the most serious fungal infections that can affect humans. These illnesses are often silent, hard to detect, and in some cases, extremely lethal—like cryptococcosis. Always treat fungal threats with the same care and attention as any parasite or virus.

Disease / Pathogen	Main Animal Host/Reservoir	Transmission
Histoplasma capsulatum – Histoplasmosis	Birds, bats (via droppings)	Inhalation of spores from droppings in caves, old buildings, or soil.
Coccidioides immitis – Coccidioidomycosis (Valley Fever)	Rodents (soil contamination)	Inhalation of airborne spores in arid, dusty regions.
**Cryptococcus neoformans* – Cryptococcosis	Pigeons (droppings)	Inhalation of spores from dried bird droppings or contaminated areas.
Sporothrix schenckii – Sporotrichosis	Cats, soil, plants	Through cat scratches or skin contact with contaminated soil/plants.
Microsporum canis / *Trichophyton* spp. – Ringworm	Dogs, cats, cattle	Direct contact with infected animals or contaminated objects (brushes, beds).

*See example below

Major Fungal Diseases Transmitted by Animals or Environment

Fungi are everywhere in nature, but some can cause disease in humans—especially in those with weakened immune systems. This table outlines key fungal infections transmitted through environmental exposure or animal contact. Proper hygiene, personal protection, and quick diagnosis are crucial for controlling their impact.

Characteristics	**Histoplasmosis**	**Valley Fever (Coccidioidomycosis)**	**Sporotrichosis**	**Ringworm (Dermatophytosis)**
Transmission / Vectors	Inhalation of spores from bird/bat droppings	Inhalation of spores from dry soil/dust	Skin injury with contaminated plant or cat scratch	Direct contact with infected animals, surfaces
Signs and Symptoms	Cough, chest pain, fever, fatigue	Cough, fever, fatigue, joint pain	Skin ulcers, nodules, lymph node swelling	Itchy, circular skin patches, hair loss
Diagnosis / Tests	Chest X-ray, antigen test, culture	Chest X-ray, serology, fungal culture	Biopsy, fungal culture	Skin scraping, Wood's lamp exam
Prevention / Prophylaxis	Avoid caves, dusty areas with droppings	Avoid dust in endemic areas, masks	Wear gloves, avoid handling stray cats	Good hygiene, treat infected animals
Treatment	Requires antifungal medication	Requires antifungal medication	Antifungals, early diagnosis essential	Antifungal creams or oral meds—consult vet/ doctor
Geographic Distribution	Americas, especially Central & South America	Southwestern U.S., Mexico, parts of LATAM	Tropical and subtropical areas	Worldwide, common in pets and humans

Disease: Cryptococcosis (*Cryptococcus neoformans*)

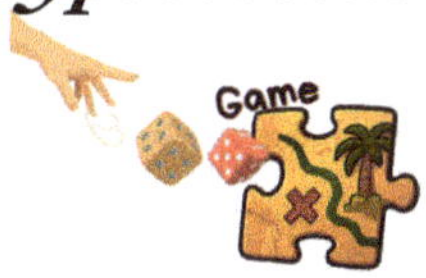

Transmission / Vectors

Infection occurs by inhaling airborne spores, especially from dried pigeon droppings or contaminated soil.

Not spread person-to-person or from animals directly.

Signs and Symptoms

Starts with cough, fever, fatigue.

Can progress to meningitis in immunocompromised individuals (HIV/AIDS), causing headache, neck stiffness, confusion, and even coma.

Diagnosis / Tests

Blood and cerebrospinal fluid (CSF) tests — antigen detection, culture, or India ink staining.

Lumbar puncture is often needed to confirm meningitis.

Prevention / Prophylaxis

Avoid areas with heavy pigeon droppings or bird roosts.

Use protective equipment when cleaning bird-infested areas.

In HIV+ patients, maintain good immune health with antiretroviral therapy.

Treatment

A doctor will confirm the diagnosis and begin the correct treatment. Do not self-medicate.

💊 Antifungal therapy.

⧗ Treatment duration depends on severity and immune status.

Geographic Distribution

● Found worldwide, especially in urban areas, regions with large bird populations, and in immunocompromised patients.

General Prevention Tips for Fungal Infections

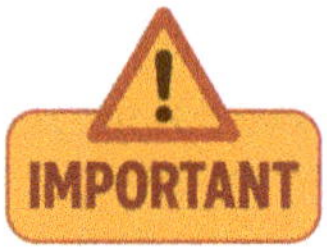

I. Avoid Contact with Animal Fungal Lesions

- Wear gloves when handling infected pets, and seek veterinary care quickly.
- Disinfect grooming tools, bedding, and toys.

II. Protect Yourself in Dusty or Contaminated Areas

- Use masks when entering areas with bird/bat droppings, caves, or old buildings.
- Avoid disturbing dry soil in endemic areas without protection.

III. Wear Gloves When Gardening

- Protect your skin from potential *Sporothrix* spores in soil, plants, or thorny bushes.
- Treat any scratches or cuts quickly.

IV. Clean Up Bird and Bat Droppings Safely

- Use PPE (gloves, mask) and avoid sweeping dry droppings —dampen surfaces first.
- Avoid storing pet food or water bowls near roosting birds.

V. Keep Immunocompromised Individuals Safe

- Limit exposure to potential fungal hotspots (e.g., pigeons, compost, dust storms).
- Use air filtration in high-risk homes or areas.

VI. Treat All Pets Promptly

- If a dog, cat, or horse shows signs of ringworm (circular bald patches), seek veterinary attention immediately.
- Treat the environment to prevent reinfection.

Fungi may be silent, invisible invaders—but with knowledge, care, and good hygiene, we can keep both our families and our furry friends safe.

Nature is amazing, and so is prevention!

These diseases highlight the importance of responsible pet ownership, including routine veterinary check-ups, vaccinations, and regular deworming to protect both animals and humans from infections.

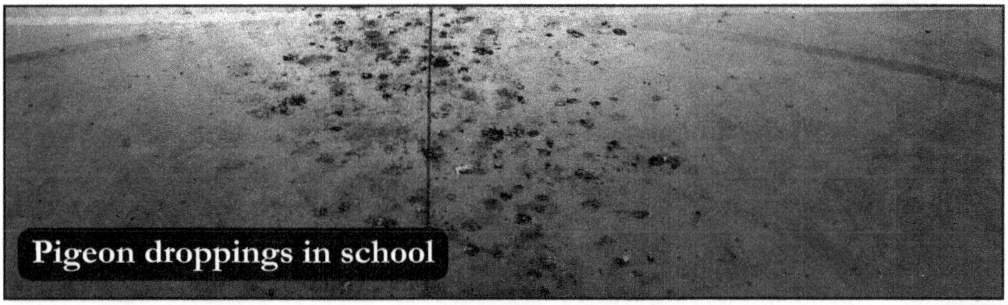

▲ **Attention – Danger:** These are pigeon droppings on a sports court where many children play and exercise daily. In situations like this, never use a broom—it can stir up fungal spores into the air. Instead, use water to safely wash the area and carry the pathogens away. Proper cleaning helps protect everyone's health.

Just as our pets require medical care, humans should also consult healthcare professionals for proper preventive treatments and medications when necessary.

Additionally, food safety is crucial—when consuming animal proteins such as beef, pork, poultry, or even fish, it is essential to cook them thoroughly.

Proper cooking eliminates many parasites and pathogens that could otherwise pose serious health risks. Avoiding raw or undercooked meats significantly reduces the chance of infection, ensuring a safer and healthier diet for you and your family.

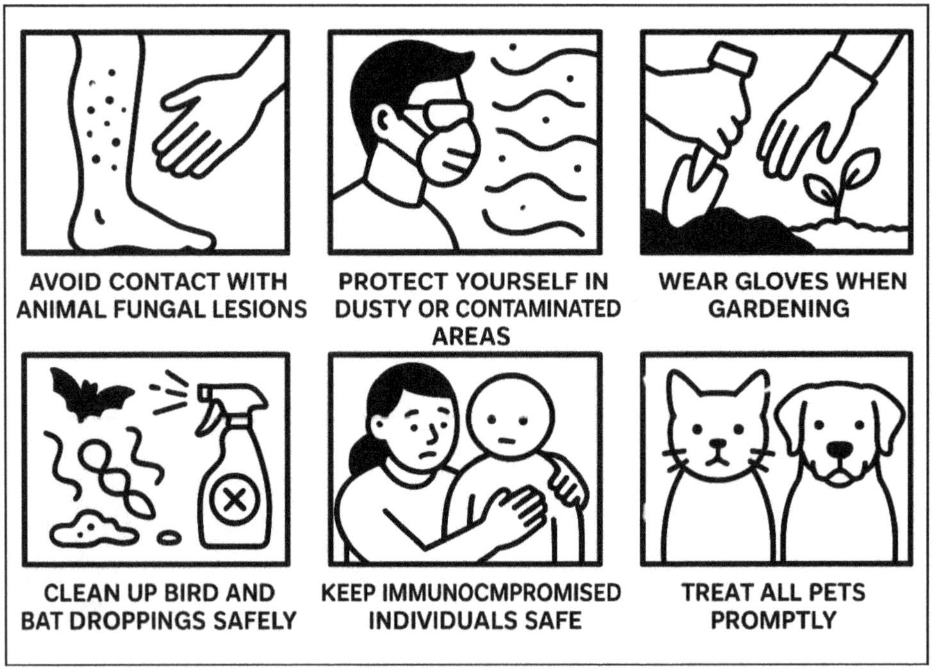
AVOID CONTACT WITH ANIMAL FUNGAL LESIONS
PROTECT YOURSELF IN DUSTY OR CONTAMINATED AREAS
WEAR GLOVES WHEN GARDENING
CLEAN UP BIRD AND BAT DROPPINGS SAFELY
KEEP IMMUNOCMPROMISED INDIVIDUALS SAFE
TREAT ALL PETS PROMPTLY

These preventive actions are essential to avoid serious fungal infections that can affect the lungs, skin, and internal organs. Without early diagnosis and protection, these diseases may lead to severe health complications — or even death. Protect yourself and others by following these simple, life-saving measures every day.

The Parasite Dice Game II

Roll the dice and start your parasite adventure!

Use a real die or a dice app on your phone to play!

First, roll the die once to choose which disease you'll face.

Then, roll again to select one of its key characteristics (like how it spreads or how to prevent it!).

Got it right? Score 10 points!

Got it wrong? Pass the die to the next player.

Who will be the best Parasite Hunter? Let the battle of brains and biology begin!

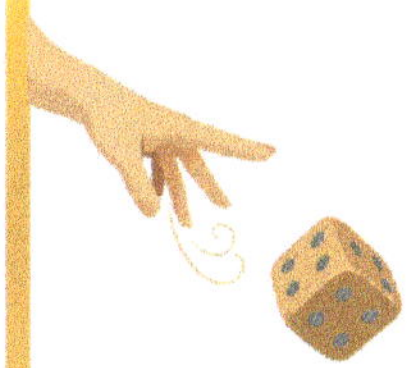

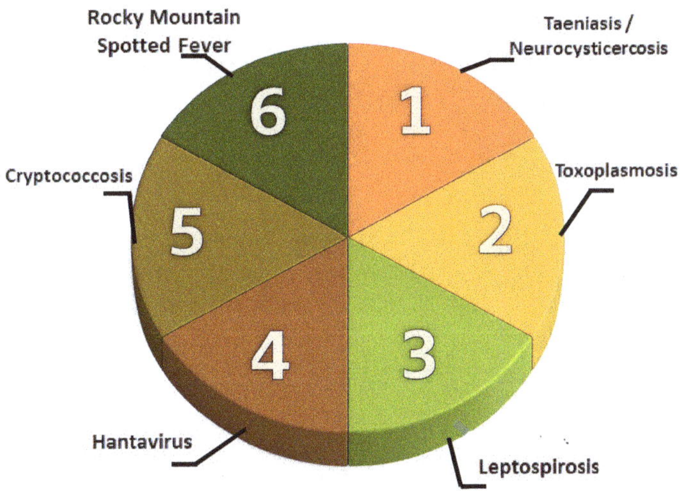

Key Characteristics to Know:

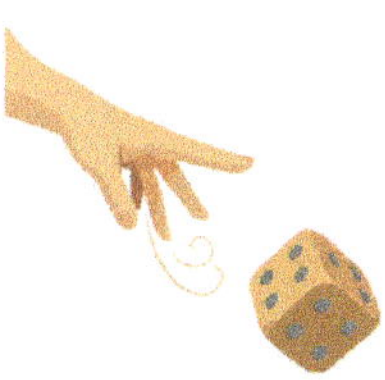

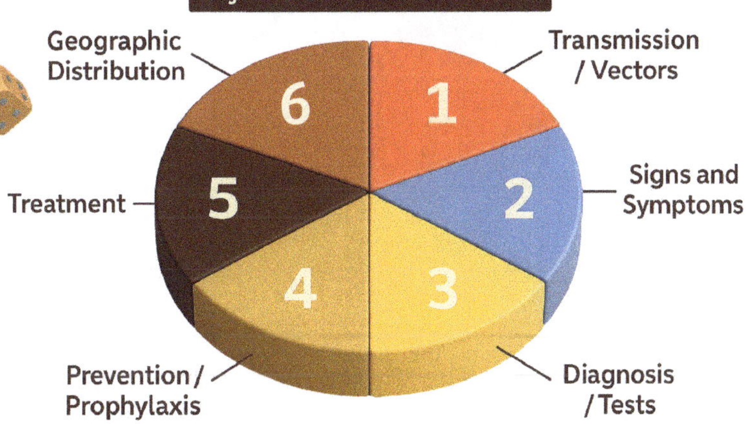

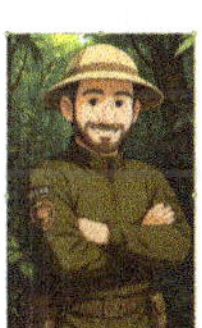

Chapter 4

Biological and Mechanical Vectors

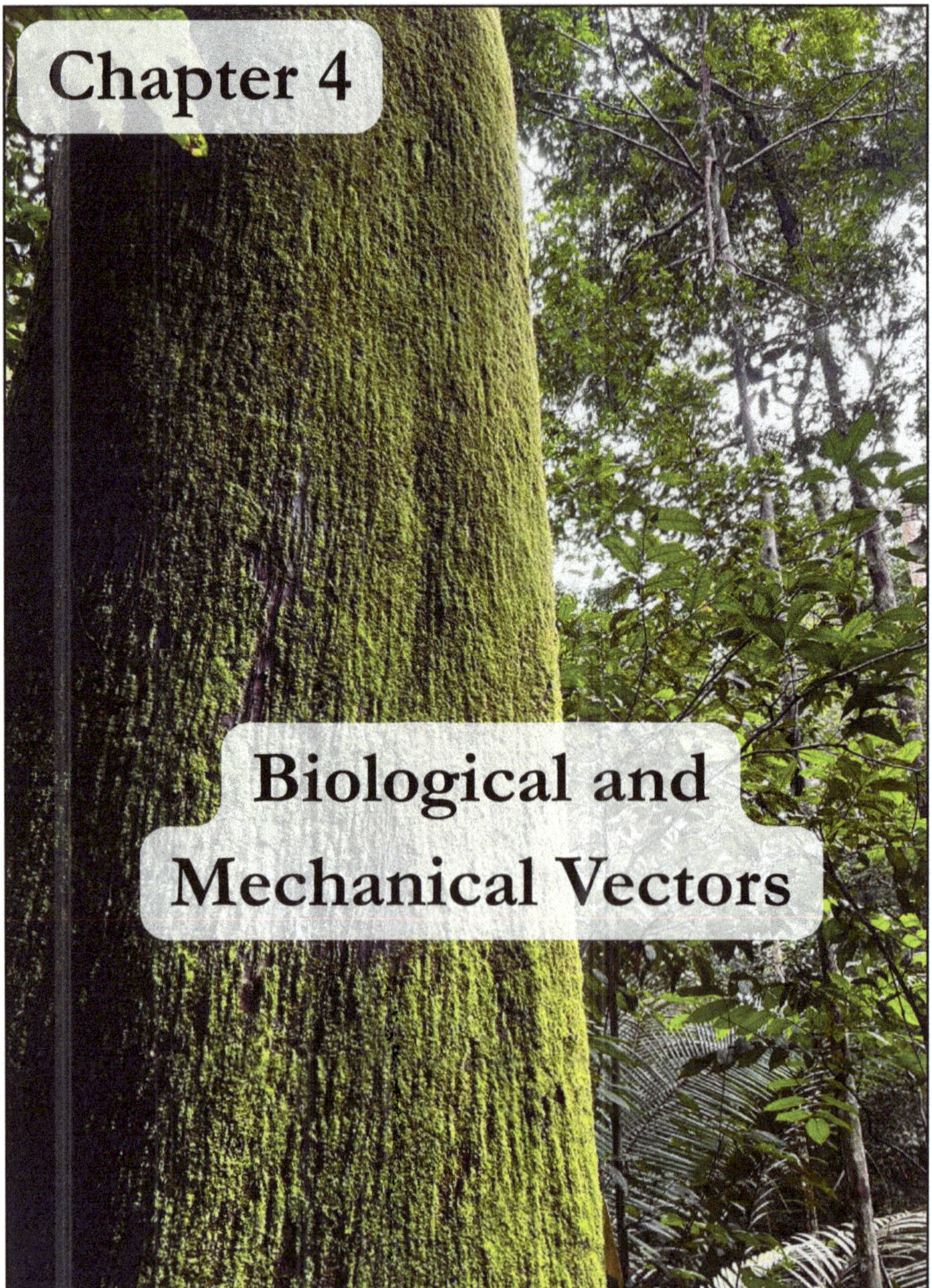

A single tree trunk deep in the Amazon rainforest. Just imagine how many tiny microorganisms live within its moss, roots, and canopy. Thousands? Millions? Over its 800-year lifespan, this tree becomes a home and food source for an entire hidden world of life.

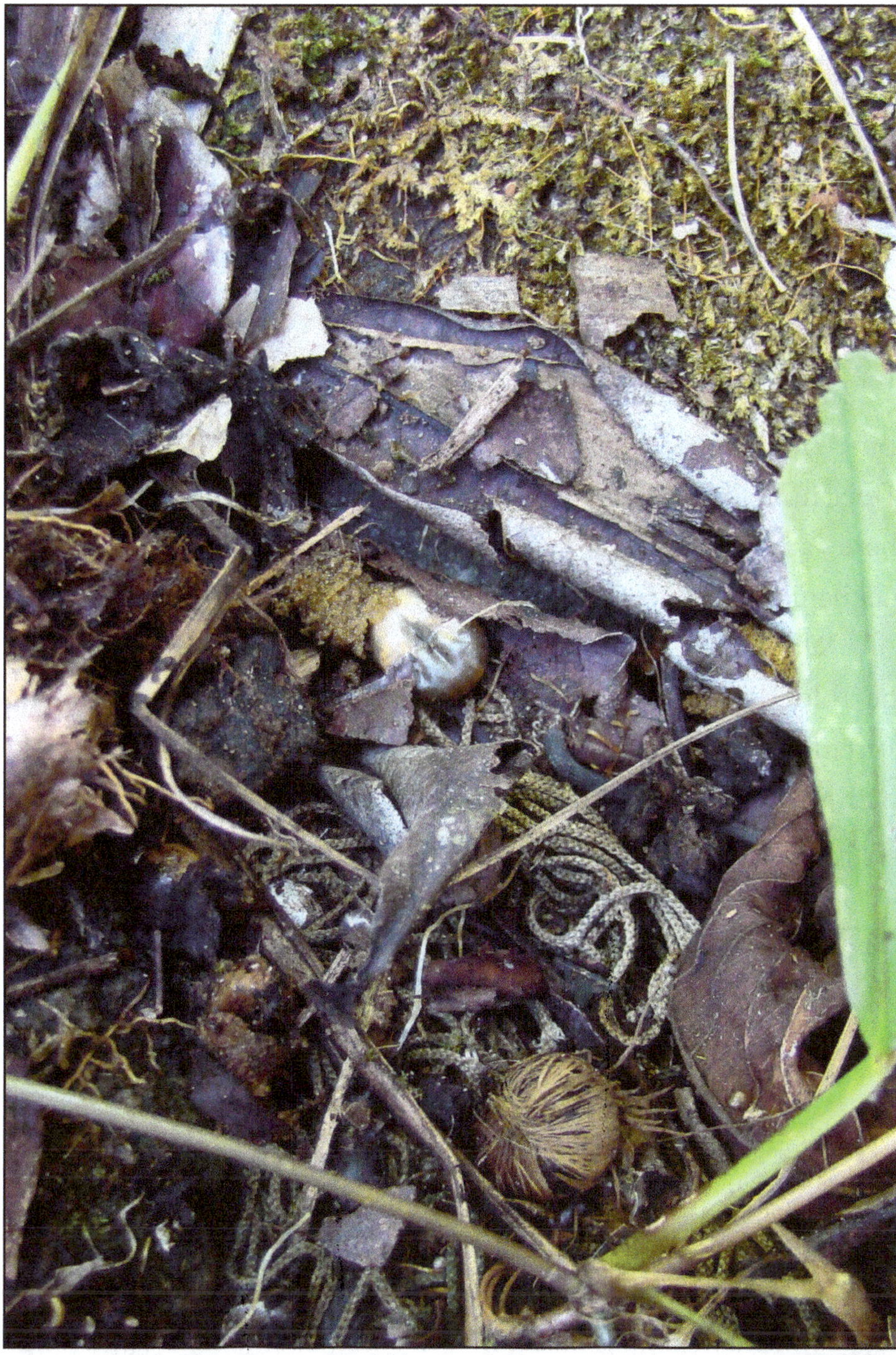

In this image, a female tick (*Amblyomma ovale*) is hiding while laying over 5,000 eggs. Did you spot her?

Tiny Transmitters of Major Diseases

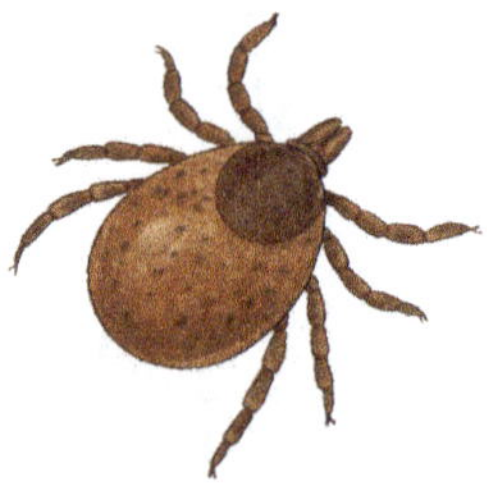

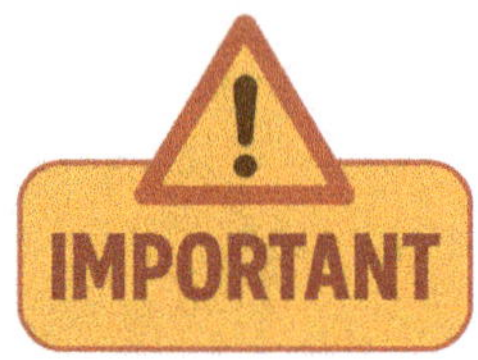
IMPORTANT

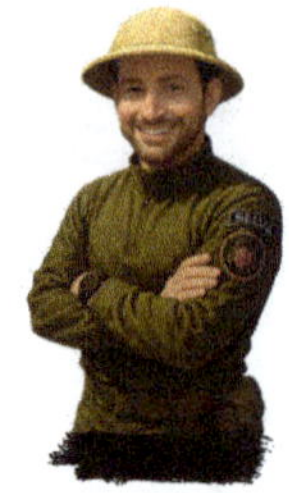

In nature, arthropods play essential roles in ecosystems, but some of them are also responsible for spreading diseases that affect humans and animals. In the world of infectious diseases, there are two main categories of vectors: biological and mechanical.

Whether it's an infected mosquito injecting parasites into the bloodstream or a fly landing on food after visiting contaminated waste, these small creatures are key players in microorganism transmission. Let's explore their differences!

Biological Vectors

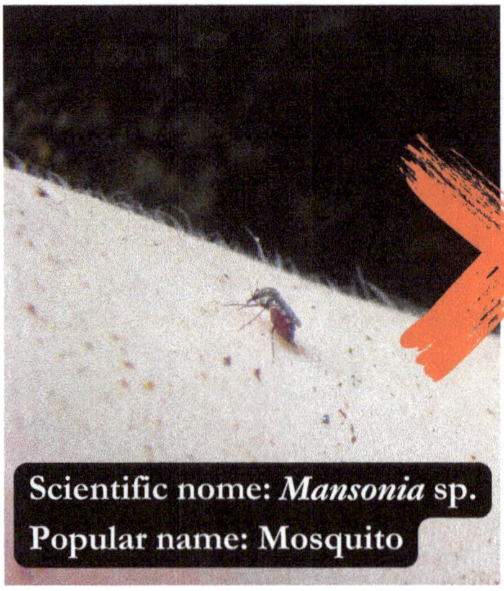
Scientific nome: *Mansonia* sp.
Popular name: Mosquito

Mechanical Vectors

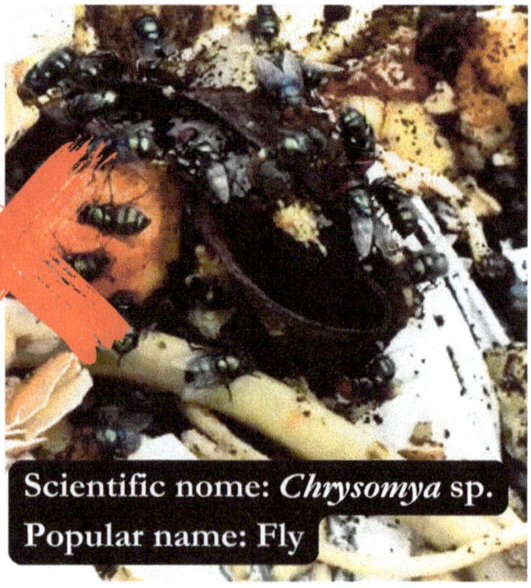
Scientific nome: *Chrysomya* sp.
Popular name: Fly

Biological Vectors

These are the main biological vectors responsible for transmitting diseases worldwide. Together, they cause millions of new cases each year. Knowing them is key to learning how to protect yourself.

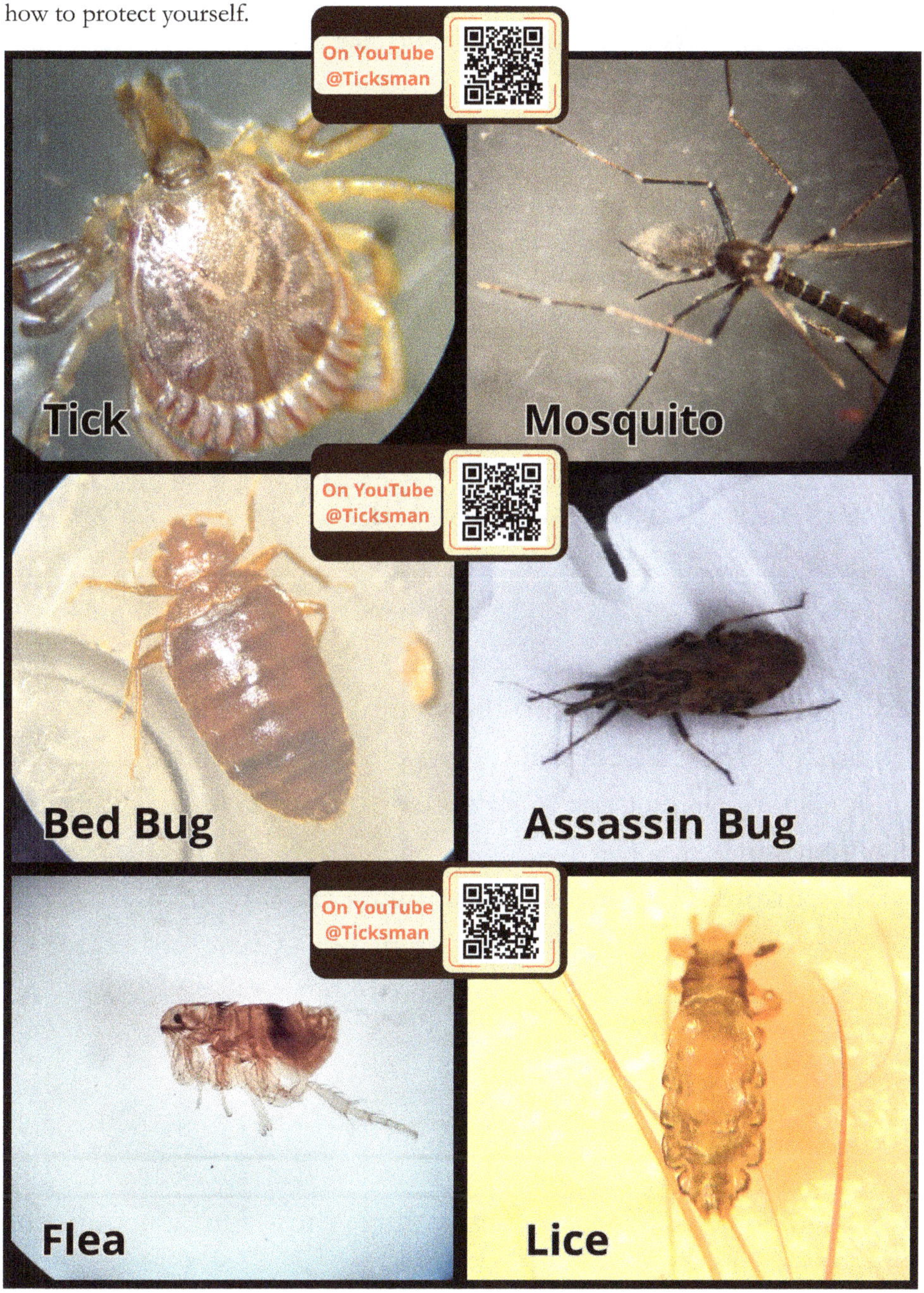

Biological Vectors: A Crucial Part of the Pathogen's Life Cycle

Biological vectors are arthropods that not only transport infectious agents but also serve as a site for their development and multiplication. These vectors are essential to the pathogen's life cycle and are directly involved in its transmission.
How does it work?

The biological vector acquires the microorganism by feeding on an infected host. After an incubation period inside its body, the pathogen becomes capable of being transmitted to another organism.

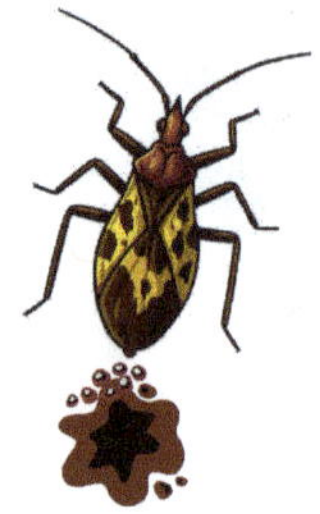

Transmission occurs through:

Saliva:

During a bite, the vector injects saliva containing the infectious agent directly into the victim's bloodstream.

- **Example I:** The female *Anopheles* spp. mosquito transmits malaria by injecting *Plasmodium* spp. sporozoites into the host's blood.
- **Example II:** The Assassin bug (*Triatoma* spp., *Rhodnius* spp. or *Panstrongylus* spp.) transmits Chagas disease by defecating near the bite site, releasing *Trypanosoma cruzi*.

Contaminated feces:

Some vectors eliminate the pathogen in their feces, and infection occurs when the person scratches the bite site and introduces the microorganism into the skin or mucous membranes.

- **Example III:** The human body louse (*Pediculus humanus humanus*) transmits epidemic typhus by excreting *Rickettsia prowazekii* near the scalp or skin.

Regurgitation:

Some vectors release pathogens along with digestive fluids while feeding.

- **Example IV:** The rat flea (*Xenopsylla cheopis*) regurgitates *Yersinia pestis*, the bacteria that cause bubonic plague, into a new host during feeding.

Biological vectors are considered highly efficient in spreading diseases because they allow the pathogen to multiply inside them before transmission.

Mechanical Vectors: Passive Carriers of Contamination

Unlike biological vectors, mechanical vectors do not participate in the pathogen's life cycle. They only transport infectious agents from one place to another passively, without allowing the microorganism to develop inside them.

How does it work?

The mechanical vector carries microorganisms on its legs, antennae, body hairs, or even on its surface, transferring them from contaminated areas to food, objects, or open wounds.

Contaminated legs:

The vector walks over feces, garbage, or infected carcasses and then steps on food or human-contact surfaces.

- **Example V:** Houseflies (*Musca domestica*) spread bacteria like *Salmonella* and *Escherichia coli* by landing on food after visiting contaminated areas.

Body contact:

The vector directly touches human mucous membranes after carrying pathogens on its body.

- **Example VI:** Cockroaches (Blattodea) can carry viruses, bacteria, and fungi on their antennae and legs, contaminating surfaces they traverse.

Wounds and accidental stings:

Some non-blood-feeding insects can transmit diseases by stinging accidentally.

- **Example VII:** Bees and wasps can introduce pathogens into a person's body if they sting after contacting contaminated organic matter.

Although less specialized than biological vectors, mechanical vectors pose a significant risk because they can carry multiple pathogens at once, contaminating food, water, and surfaces.

PREVENTION IS KEY!

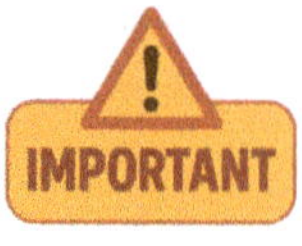

Small but Powerful

Distinguishing between biological and mechanical vectors is essential for understanding disease transmission and taking protective measures.

- Biological Vectors actively participate in the disease cycle and transmit pathogens through saliva, feces, or regurgitation.

- Mechanical Vectors merely carry pathogens on their bodies, spreading contamination to food and surfaces.
- Using repellents and mosquito nets reduces exposure to biological vectors.
- Pest control and proper hygiene help prevent mechanical vectors.

By better understanding these tiny transmitters, we can adopt more effective measures to combat the diseases they spread and protect our health!

Preventing arthropod-borne diseases requires targeted strategies for each type of vector.

Below are detailed prevention methods for ticks, fleas, bed bugs, assassin bugs, mosquitoes, and lice:

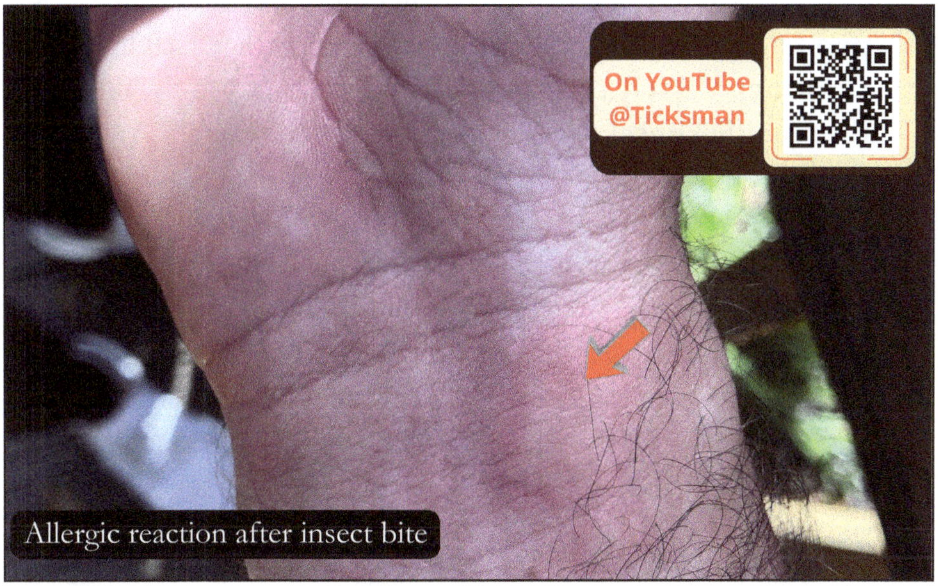

In this image, we see the author's immune system reacting to substances injected by a mosquito vector during feeding. To produce eggs, female mosquitoes require nutrient-rich blood. During hematophagy (blood feeding), they regurgitate saliva containing anticoagulants, vasodilators, anesthetics, and other molecules that help them feed unnoticed. If the mosquito is carrying pathogens, this is the moment when disease transmission to humans can occur.

Ticks: Silent and Dangerous

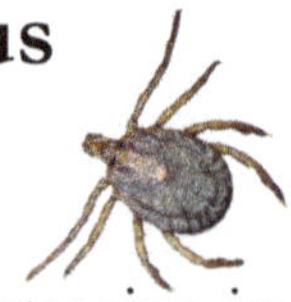

There are nearly a thousand different tick species in the world (930), and while only a small number prefer human blood, most feed on wild and domestic animals. Stay alert—if a tick remains attached for more than 4 hours, it may transmit dangerous pathogens.

- **Avoid Tick-Infested Areas:** Steer clear of wooded and brushy regions with tall grass and leaf litter.
- **Protective Clothing:** Wear long-sleeved shirts and long pants tucked into socks to minimize skin exposure.
- **Use Tick Repellents:** Apply EPA-registered repellents containing DEET or picaridin on exposed skin. Treat clothing and gear with products containing 0.5% permethrin. Attention: Always ask for medical advice.
- **Conduct Tick Checks:** After outdoor activities, thoroughly check your body and clothing for ticks. Promptly remove any attached ticks with fine-tipped tweezers.
- **Yard Maintenance:** Keep lawns mowed, remove leaf litter, and create a tick-safe zone around your home by placing a barrier of wood chips or gravel between lawns and wooded areas.

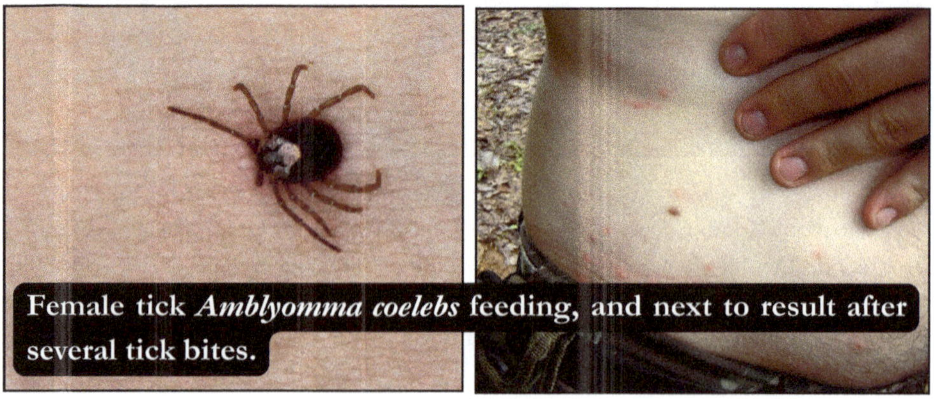

Female tick *Amblyomma coelebs* feeding, and next to result after several tick bites.

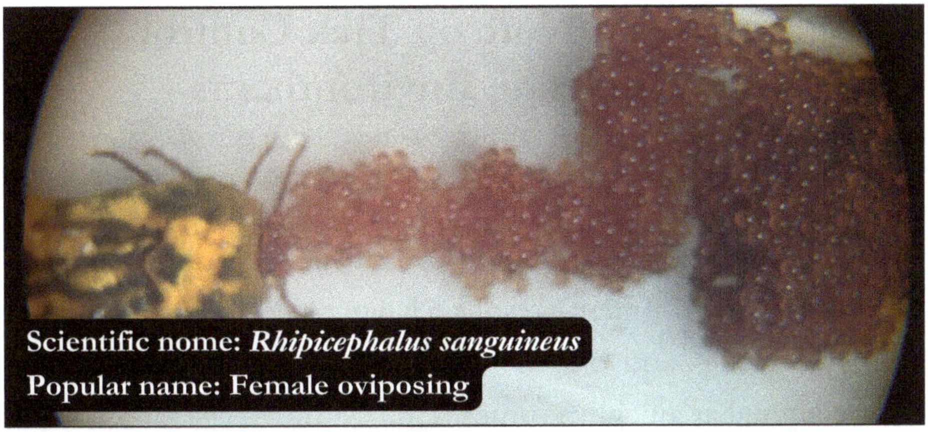
Scientific nome: *Rhipicephalus sanguineus*
Popular name: Female oviposing

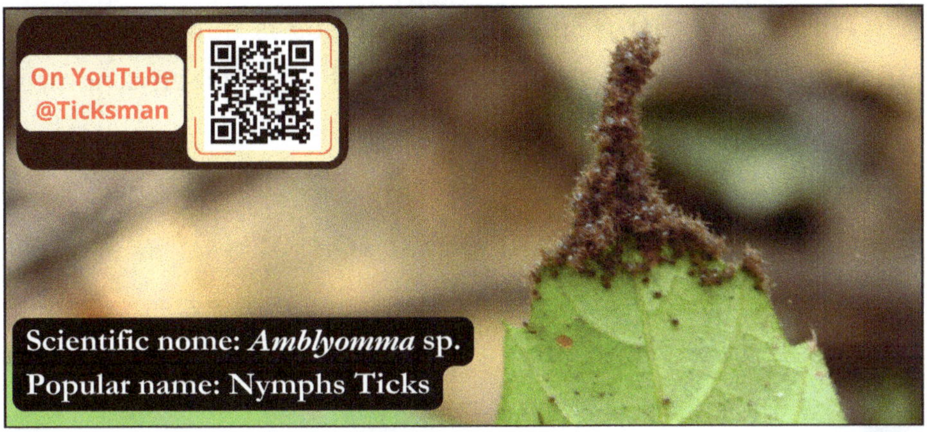
On YouTube
@Ticksman
Scientific nome: *Amblyomma* sp.
Popular name: Nymphs Ticks

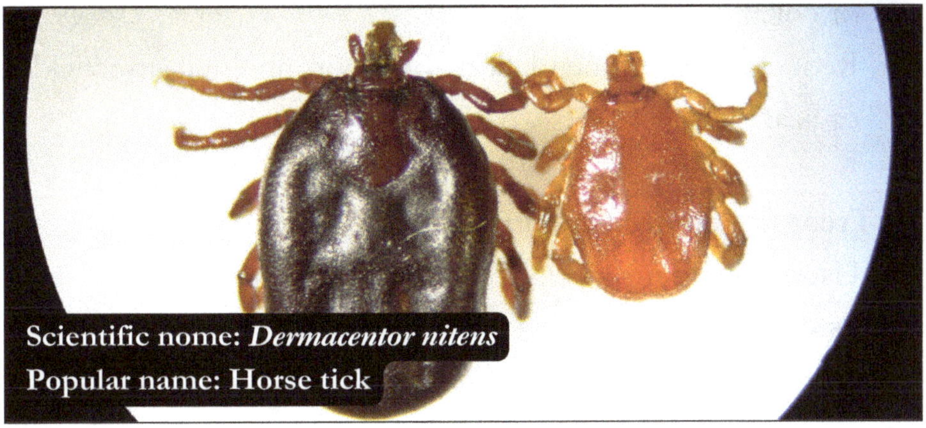

Here we see the tick's life cycle: a female laying about 3,000 eggs, larvae waiting at the tip of a leaf for their first host, and finally, an engorged female beside an adult male. The timing and duration of the cycle vary by species and region—but one thing's for sure: within a year, many new ticks will emerge.

Important Note on Tick Control in Domestic Environments

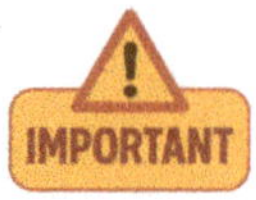

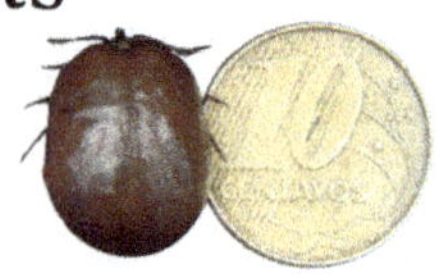

Did you know that about 95% of ticks on domestic dogs live in the environment—especially in places where your pet sleeps or rests—and only 5% are found attached and feeding on the animal at any given time?

This means that treating only your dog is not enough. For effective tick control, both the animal and its environment must be addressed simultaneously.

Here's what you need to do:

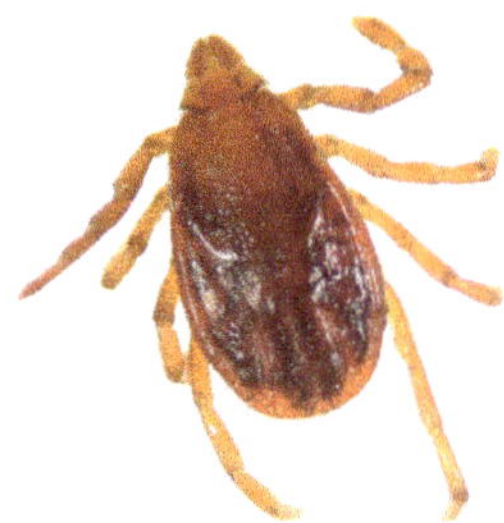

I. Consult a veterinarian:

- Ask for the best tick treatment for your pet (oral, topical, or collar).
- Request a recommendation for environmental insecticides or acaricides.

II. Treat the environment properly:

- Use a diluted insecticide in water as directed

Focus on areas like:

- Dog beds - Attention: Do not play inside human houses
- Cracks in the floor or walls
- Yard, kennel, or shaded areas where your pet spends time

III. Follow this tick control schedule:

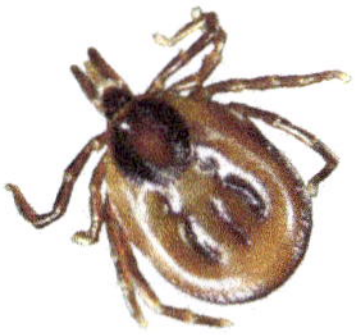

- Day 0 – First environmental application
- Day 15 – Second application
- Day 30 – Third application
- Day 45 – Fourth application
- Day 60 – Final application

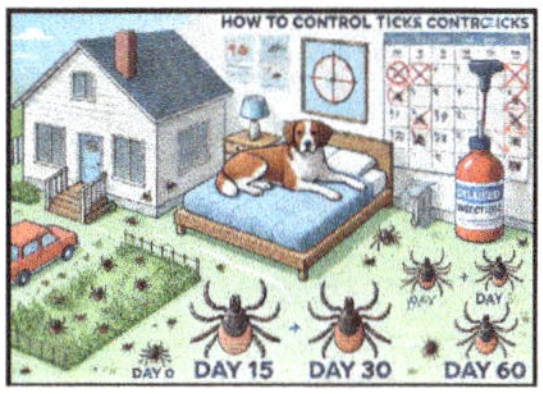

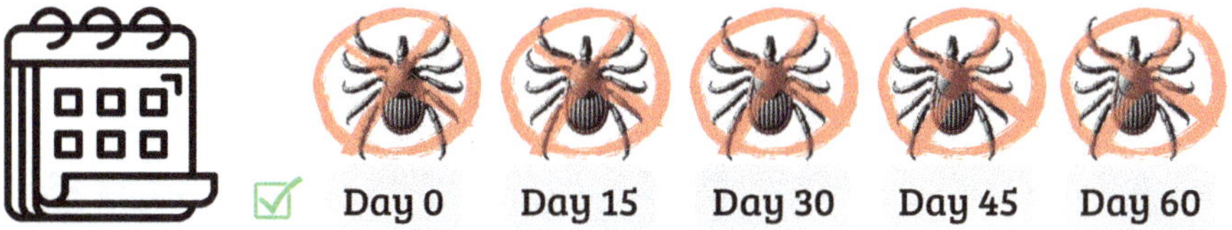

By following this treatment method, you'll achieve highly effective control of ticks on your pet. And if fleas, jiggers (*Tunga penetrans*), or mange mites are also present, there's a good chance they'll be eliminated too. This keeps your pet protected and parasite-free for an extended period.

The author inspecting a dollhouse-turned-doghouse in the Atlantic Forest region of Peruíbe, São Paulo, Brazil. Could ticks, fleas, or jiggers (*Tunga penetrans*) be hiding inside this cozy shelter?

Why is this important?

- Ticks can transmit serious diseases to pets and humans.
- Some species develop resistance to chemical treatments, so following the full environmental protocol is key to breaking the cycle.

Consistent control measures can lead to nearly 100% eradication of ticks from your home and pet environment.

When in doubt, always seek guidance from a veterinarian.

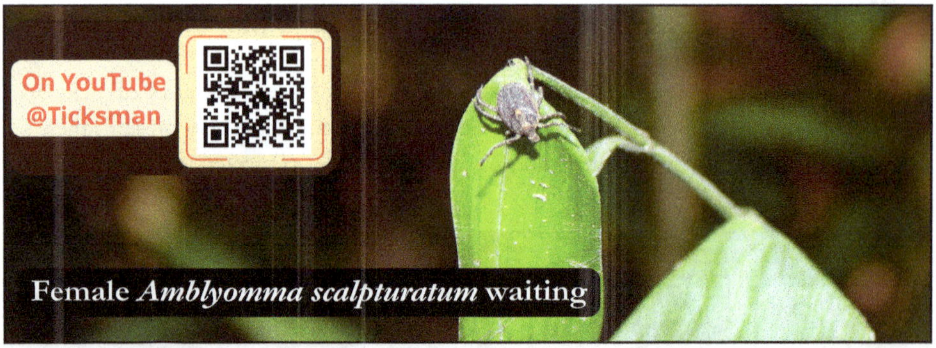

Female *Amblyomma scalpturatum* waiting

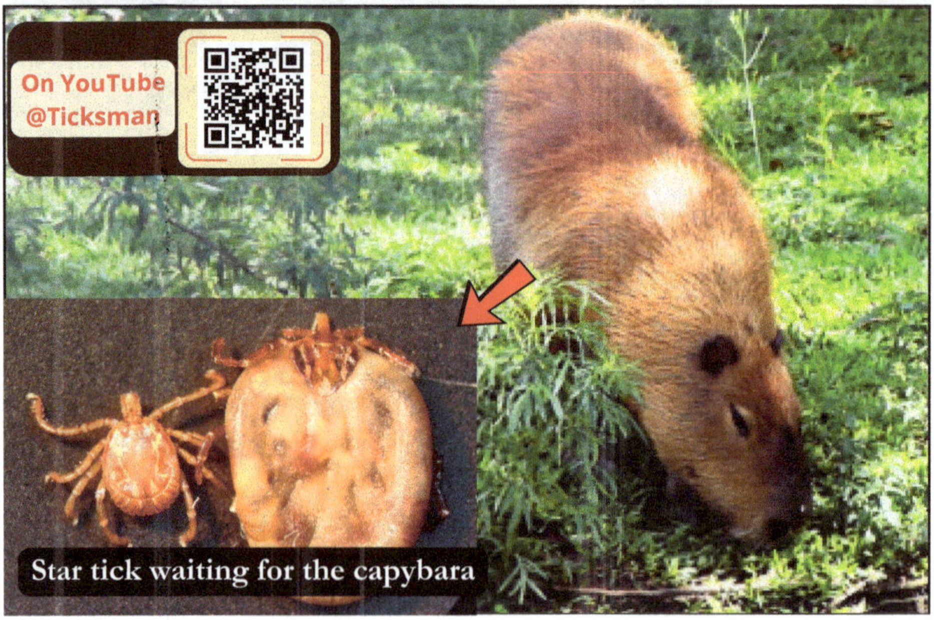

Star tick waiting for the capybara

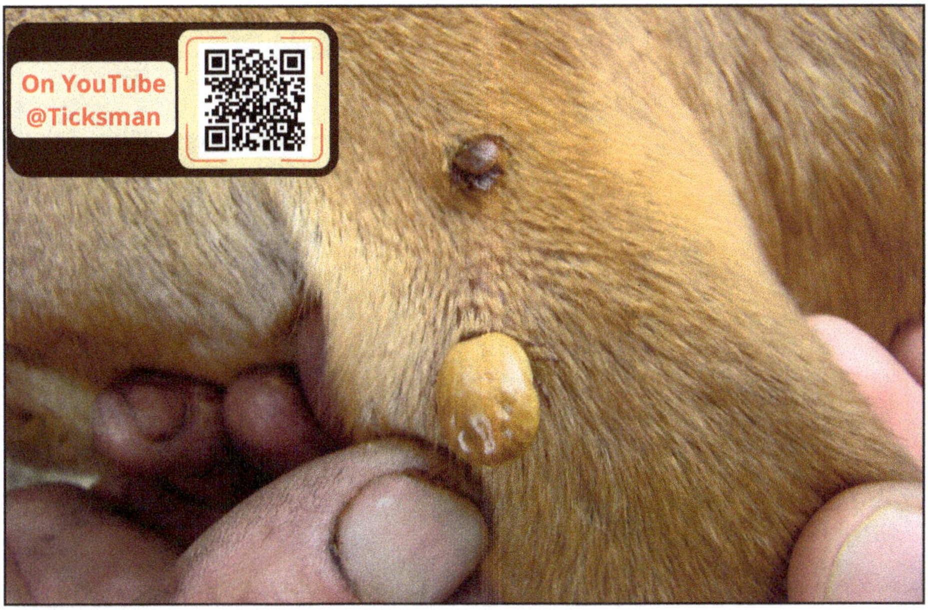

Two female and one male *Amblyomma ovale* ticks, commonly found on dogs in rural areas that roam through Amazonian forests. Females can remain attached and feed on the host's blood for up to seven days.

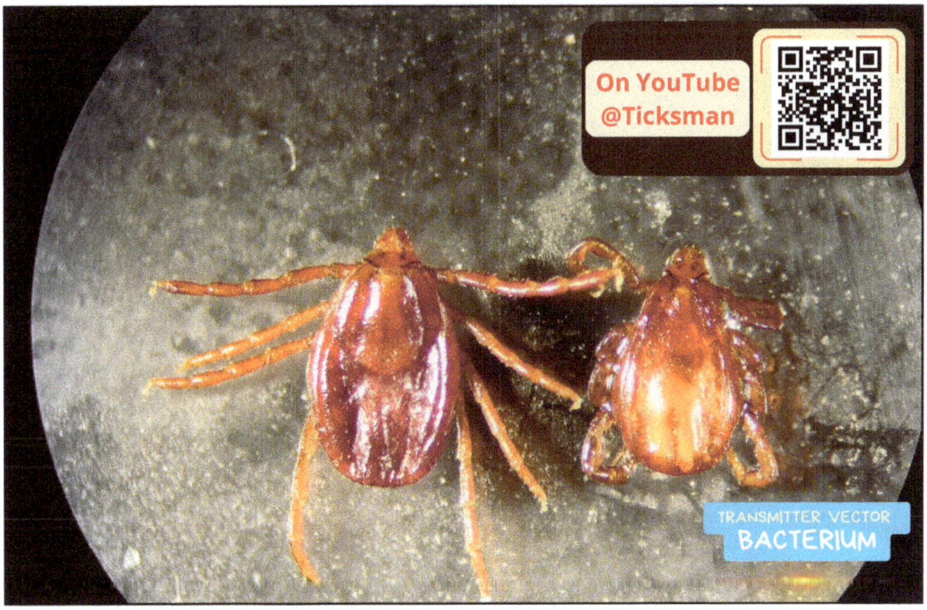

From left to right: Female and male *Rhipicephalus sanguineus* ticks photographed under magnification. This is the most common tick species found on dogs in urban areas of South America. A nidicolous tick that thrives in environments where dogs live and sleep.

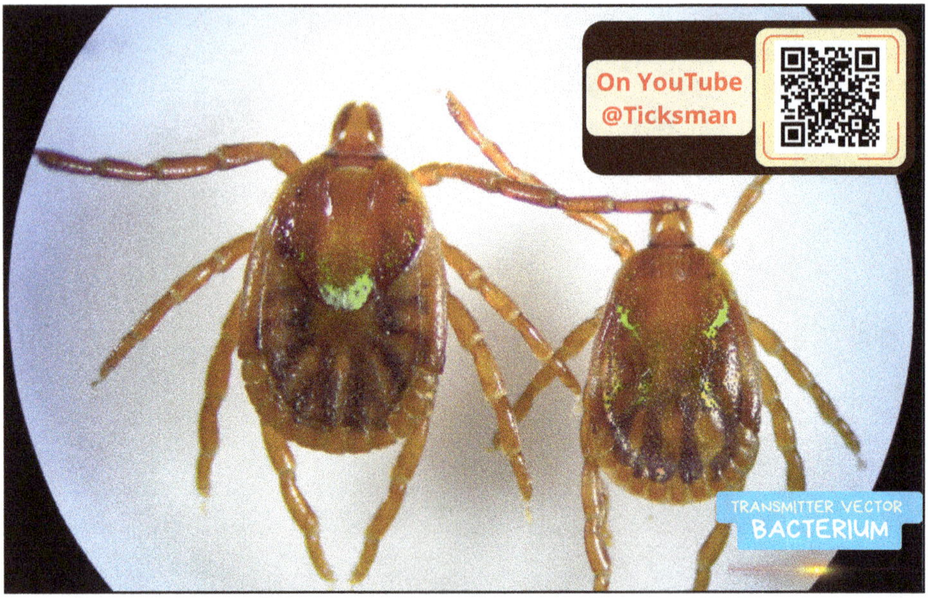

Ticks photographed under a stereomicroscope in the laboratory, highlighting morphological characteristics used for species identification. In this species (*Amblyomma ovale*), the distinctive shiny ornamentation on the scutum is a key diagnostic feature.

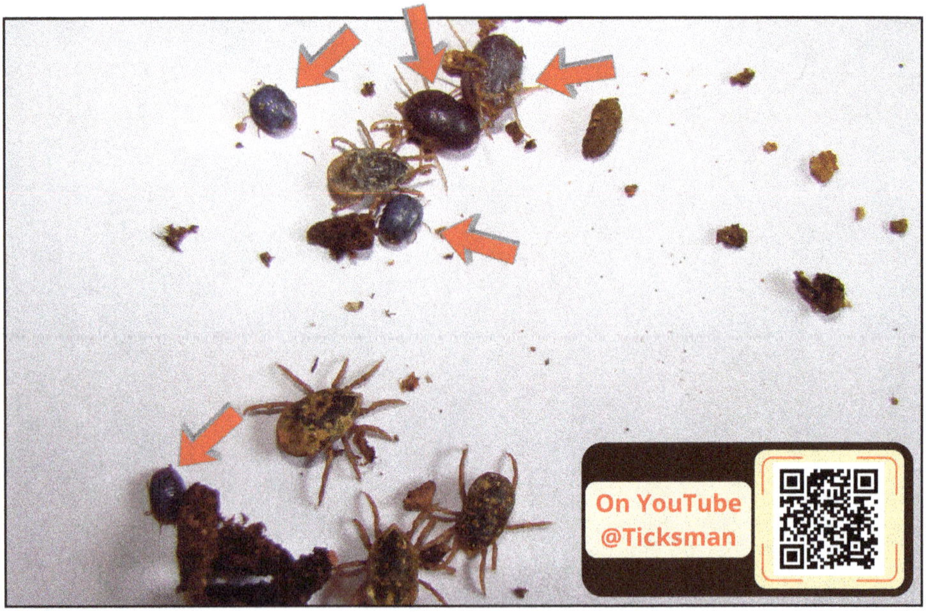

Immature stages of *Nothoaspis amazoniensis* ticks (larvae and nymphs) engorged with blood after feeding on bats in Amazonian caves. Larger adult ticks can also be seen nearby.

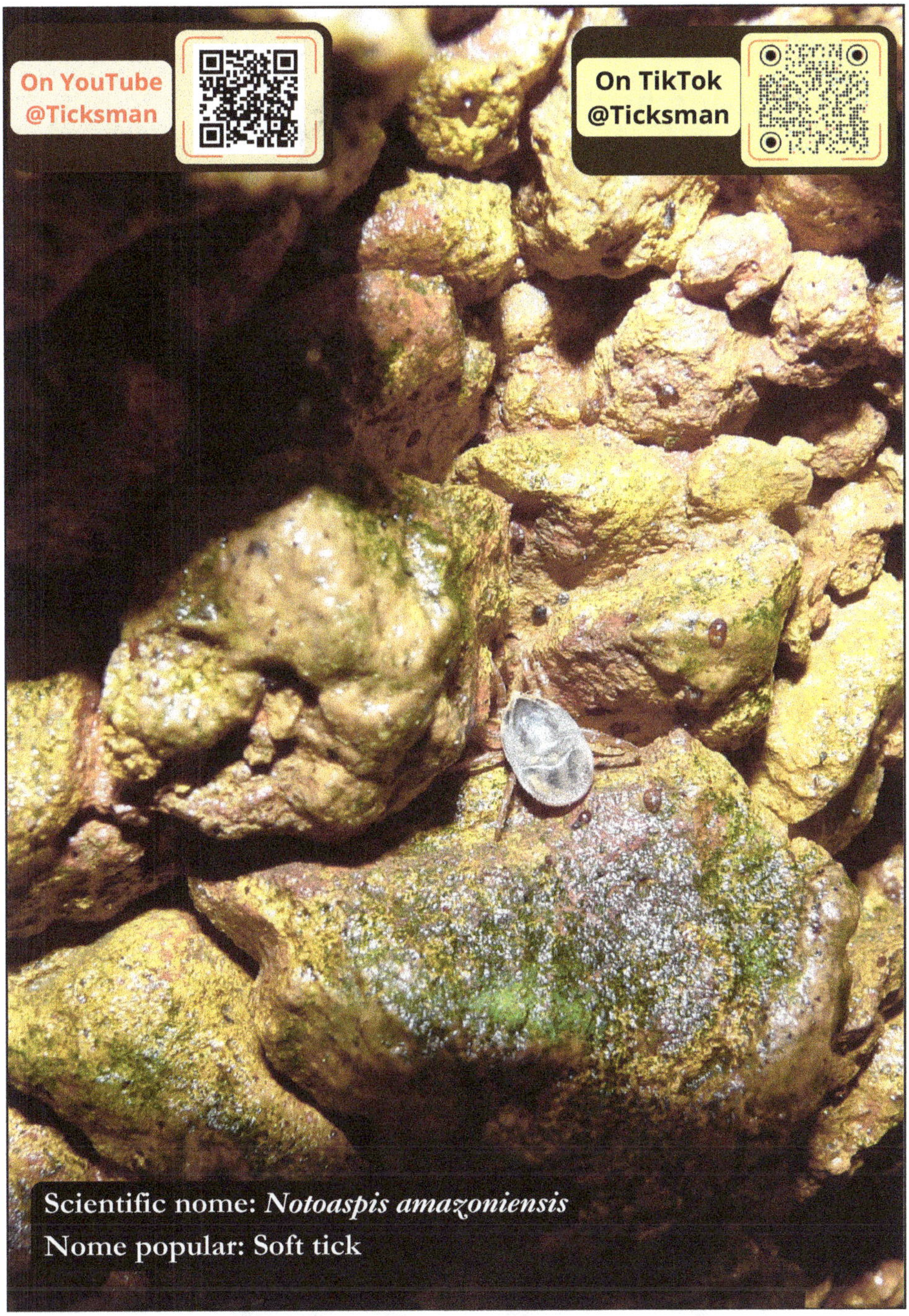
On YouTube
@Ticksman
On TikTok
@Ticksman
Scientific nome: *Notoaspis amazoniensis*
Nome popular: Soft tick

An adult *Nothoaspis amazoniensis* on a rock surface inside a cave deep in the Amazon rainforest. It is likely searching for a crevice or structure within the rock to hide and await a potential host.

Wings of Danger: The Secret Lives of Mosquitoes and Sandflies

Imagine an insect so small you can barely see it in the dark... but with one bite, it can change your life forever.

Some bring fever, others bring fatigue, and some carry silent parasites that stay hidden in your body for months—or even years.

Welcome to the mysterious world of mosquitoes and their lesser-known cousins, the phlebotomine sandflies—both champions of stealth and masters of parasitic delivery.

Why Should You Care?

These insects are the leading transmitters of some of the most widespread and dangerous tropical diseases on Earth.

They carry and transmit diseases such as:

- Malaria (*Plasmodium* spp.) – from *Anopheles* mosquitoes
- Dengue, Zika, Yellow Fever, and Chikungunya – from Aedes mosquitoes
- Leishmaniasis – from Phlebotomine sandflies.

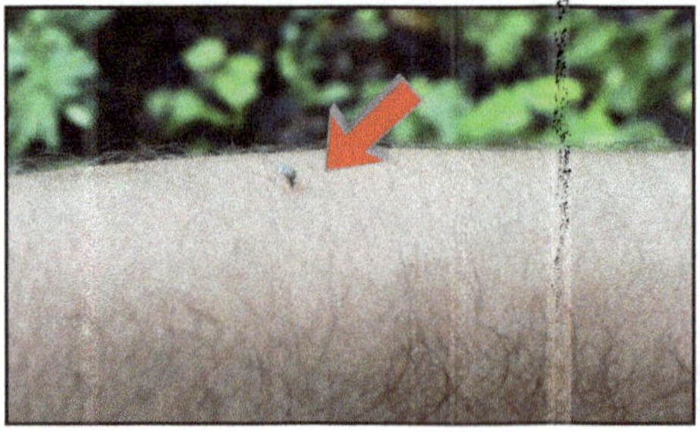

Female mosquito in the Amazon rainforest caught on the author's arm, attempting to feed on his blood.

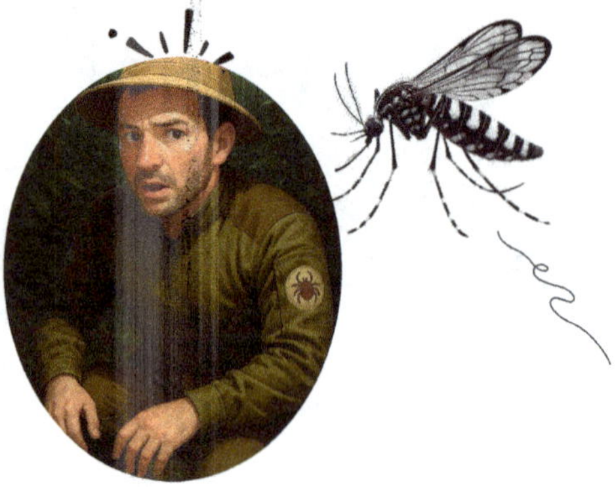

Each of these diseases can cause serious illness, disability, or death—and many thrive in urban areas, rural villages, and even deep in tropical forests.

How to Spot the Enemy (Biology & Behavior)

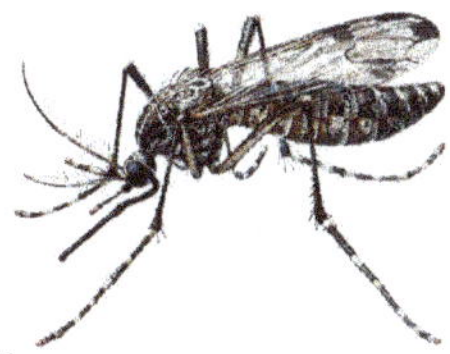

Mosquitoes:

- Only females bite—they need blood to produce eggs.
- Breeding occurs in standing water: puddles, buckets, tires, drains, flower pots.
- Active mostly at dusk, dawn, or night (depends on species).
- Life cycle: egg → larva → pupa → adult, usually within 7–14 days.

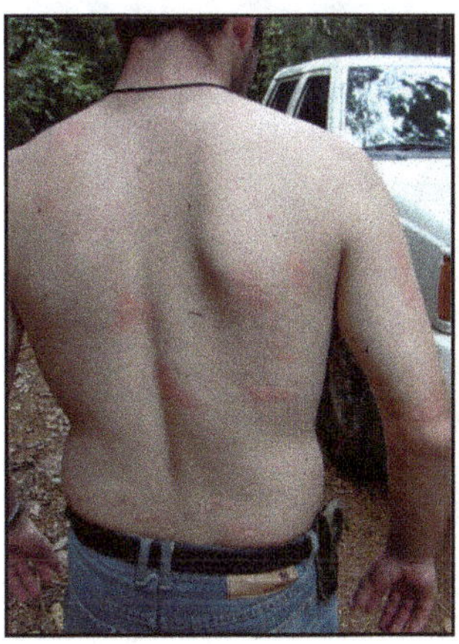

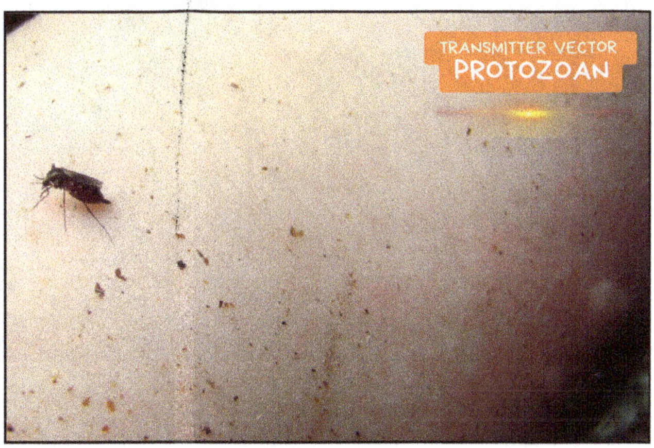

Some mosquito species around the world adapt to living near humans and develop a preference for human blood. In the first image, the author's back shows multiple bites from female *Anopheles darlingi*, which led to his first malaria infection in the Amazon. Beside it, another female mosquito is feeding — a vital step to produce eggs for the next generation. The takeaway: without blood, whether human or animal, there are no diseases — and no mosquitoes.

Sandflies (Phlebotomines):

- Tiny and silent—often mistaken for specks of dust.
- Breed in organic matter like chicken droppings, pig pens, decaying leaves, or bat guano in caves.
- Active mostly at night, and their bite can go unnoticed.
- Life cycle: egg → 4 larval stages → pupa → adult.

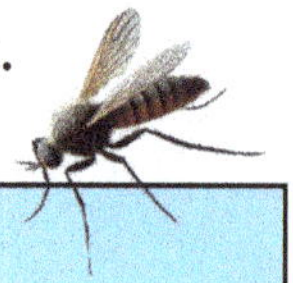

In this image, we see a rural storage house used to keep animal feed such as corn. However, the dense Amazon rainforest can be observed in the background — a natural habitat for native Phlebotomine sandflies. During a visit to this property in 2007 to collect leishmaniasis vectors, hundreds of female sandflies were captured using traps, some of them infected. Unfortunately, the farm owners tested positive for the disease. As our team included medical professionals, the individuals were promptly diagnosed and referred for treatment in the nearest town, located approximately 56 miles (90 km) away, in Assis Brasil, Acre, Brazil.

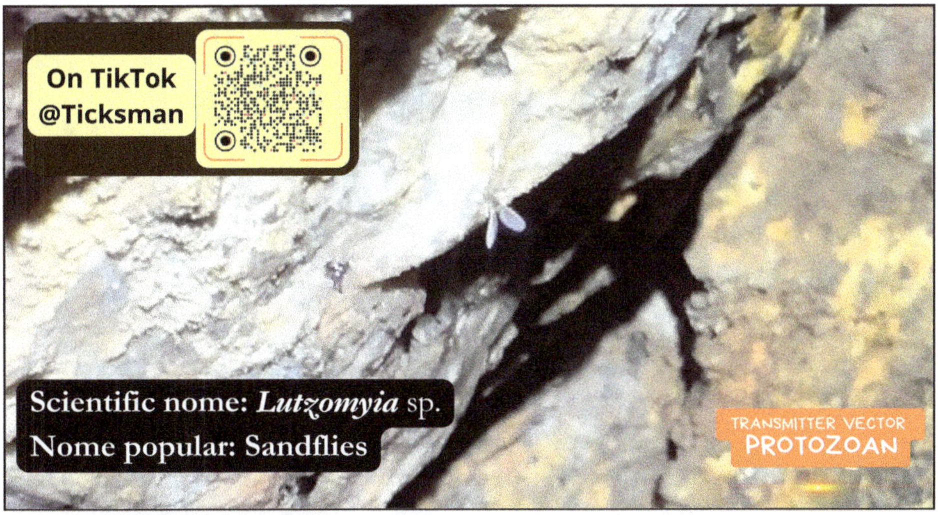
On TikTok
@Ticksman
Scientific nome: *Lutzomyia* sp.
Nome popular: Sandflies
TRANSMITTER VECTOR
PROTOZOAN

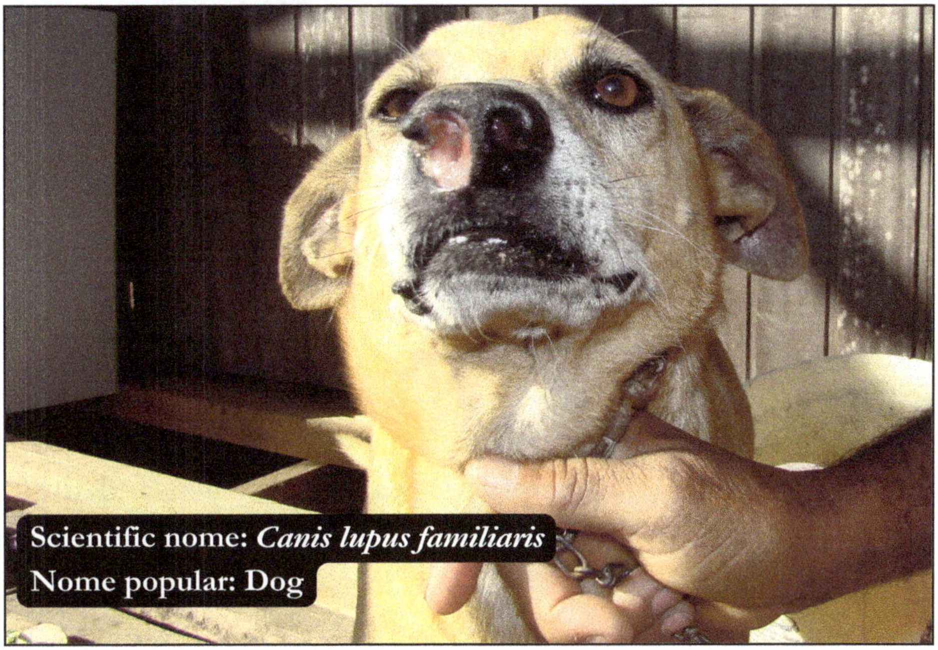
Scientific nome: *Canis lupus familiaris*
Nome popular: Dog

This dog is from the same rural region near the town of Assis Brasil, Acre, Brazil — an area with a high incidence of Leishmania. Unfortunately, dogs in this region are also commonly affected by the disease. Nasal lesion in a dog caused by cutaneous leishmaniasis. Phlebotomine sandflies, the vectors of this disease, can bite an infected dog and ingest the parasite. After a few days, if the same sandfly bites a human, it can transmit the Leishmania parasite, leading to human infection. Dogs are important reservoirs in the urban and rural transmission cycle.

Your Personal Protection Plan: How to Defeat the Winged Parasite Carriers

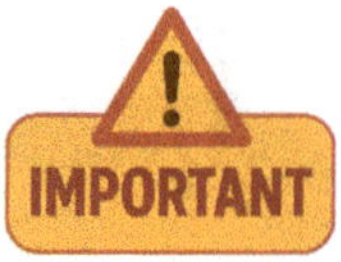

1. Eliminate Breeding Sites

- Remove standing water from containers, tires, and flowerpots every 3 days.
- Clean out gutters, cover water tanks, and fill unused holes in the ground.
- Clean up animal feces and organic waste—especially if you live near chickens, pigs, or caves.

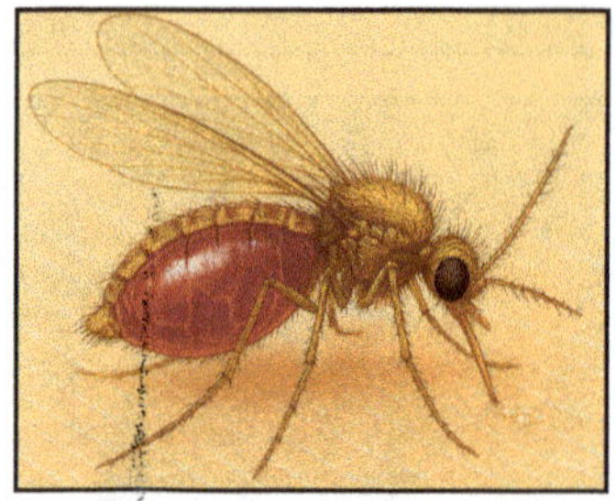

2. Create a Fortress Around You

- Install window and door screens.
- Use bed nets, especially in sleeping areas near forests or rural regions.
- Sleep under insecticide-treated nets (ITNs) in endemic zones.
- In regions where malaria is endemic, for example, avoid areas near rivers, dams and swamps at dawn and dusk, when female mosquitoes are most active.

3. Repel and Protect

- Apply EPA-registered repellents (DEET, picaridin, IR3535) to exposed skin. For children, always use repellents indicated for children (to avoid allergic reactions).
- Wear long sleeves, long pants, and socks when outside.
- Treat clothes with permethrin for extra defense.

4. Use Indoor Defenses

- Use mosquito coils, vaporizers, and insecticide sprays at night.
- Encourage use of ceiling fans—they disrupt flying patterns of light insects.

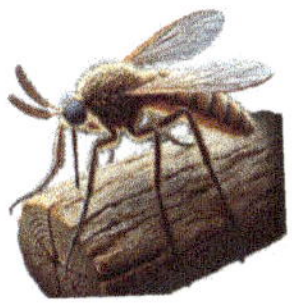

5. Control Around Pets and Animals

- Keep animal shelters clean and dry.
- Avoid allowing chickens or pigs to sleep close to your home.
- Regularly remove waste, feathers, or decaying vegetation.

6. Community Counts

- Join or organize neighborhood clean-up days.
- Educate others about mosquito and sandfly breeding grounds.
- Advocate for spraying programs and public sanitation projects.

Fun Fact: Mosquitoes are Ancient Travelers

Did you know that mosquitoes have been on Earth for over 200 million years? They were here before the dinosaurs went extinct, and they've adapted to every continent except Antarctica.

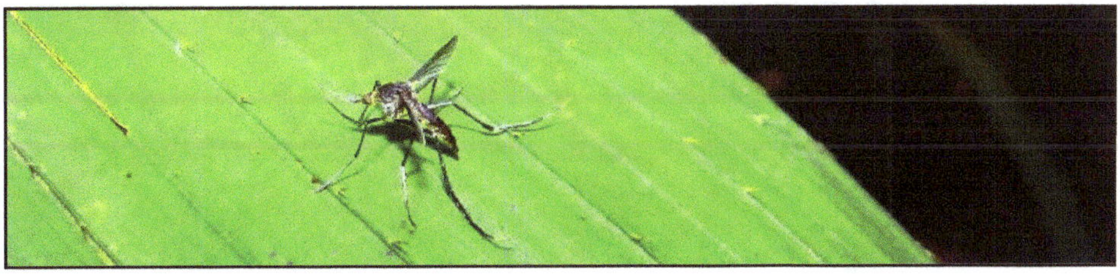

Sandflies, too, are prehistoric—some have even been found fossilized in amber!

A Note for Brave Parasite Hunters

These tiny fliers may look harmless—but one bite can carry thousands of microscopic invaders.

By knowing how they live, where they breed, and what they fear, we take control of our health, our homes, and our future.

Let's send the message: "Not in my backyard!"
Together, we can keep our skies clear and our nights bite-free.

Curiosity Note: Natural Ways to Defeat Mosquitoes

Did you know that in Disney World®, they use plants to attract dragonflies? These elegant insects lay their eggs in water, and when the larvae hatch—guess what? They become voracious predators of mosquito larvae!

In parts of Central America, people have gone even further: they introduce parasitic worm larvae and microscopic organisms into standing water to consume mosquito larvae before they can grow wings. In South America, citronella candles are used to repel adult mosquitoes with their strong scent.

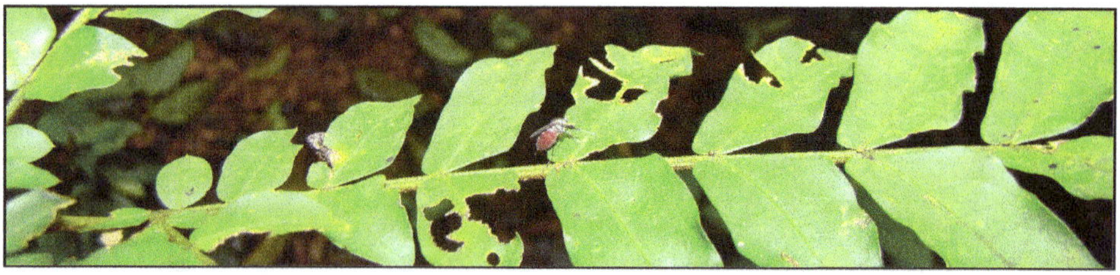

And in certain traditional cultures, people stick cloves into lemons to create a natural repellent that fills the air with mosquito-deterring aroma.

There are so many creative solutions around the world to fight these tiny disease-spreading flyers.

What about you? Do you know any other effective mosquito control trick that the world should hear about?

Share your tip on the author's social media—and maybe your idea will be featured in the next edition!

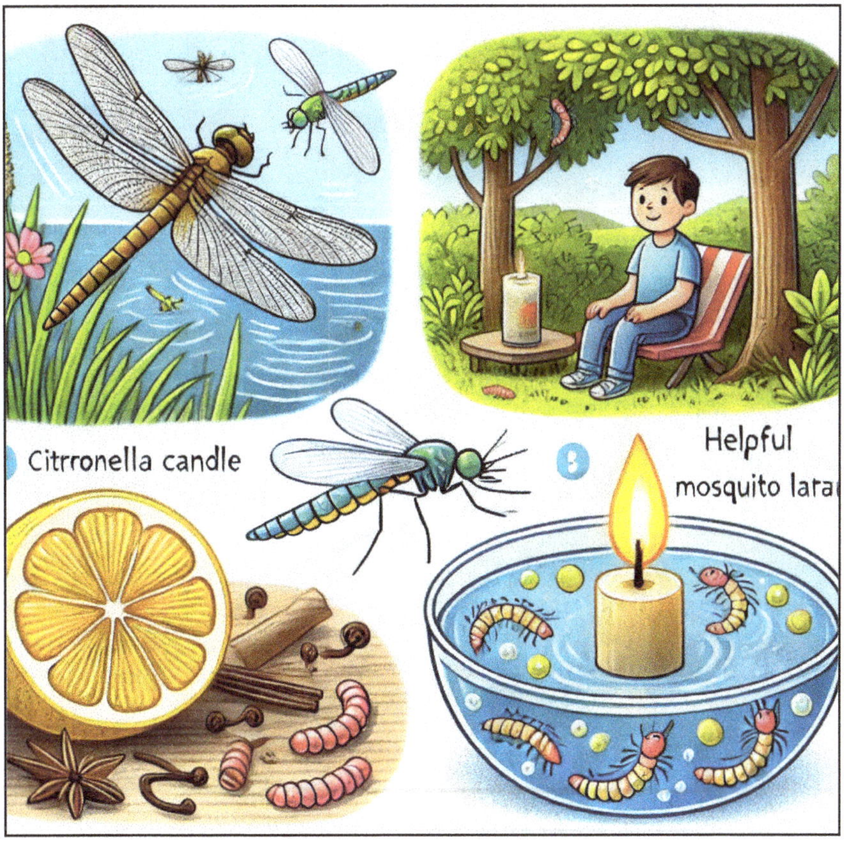

Natural mosquito control methods: dragonflies, citronella, clove-studded lemons, and helpful water organisms. Images created by artificial intelligence.

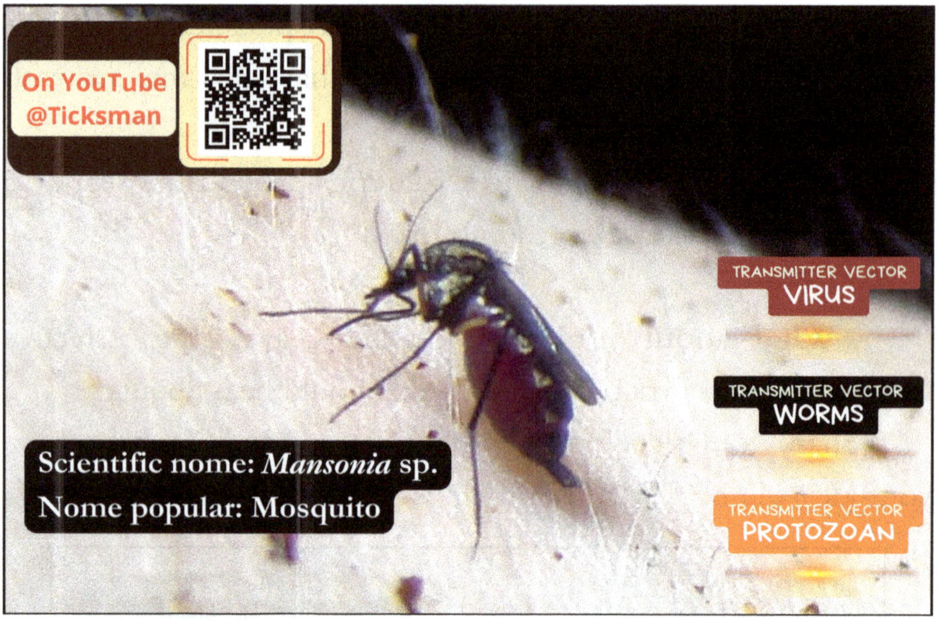

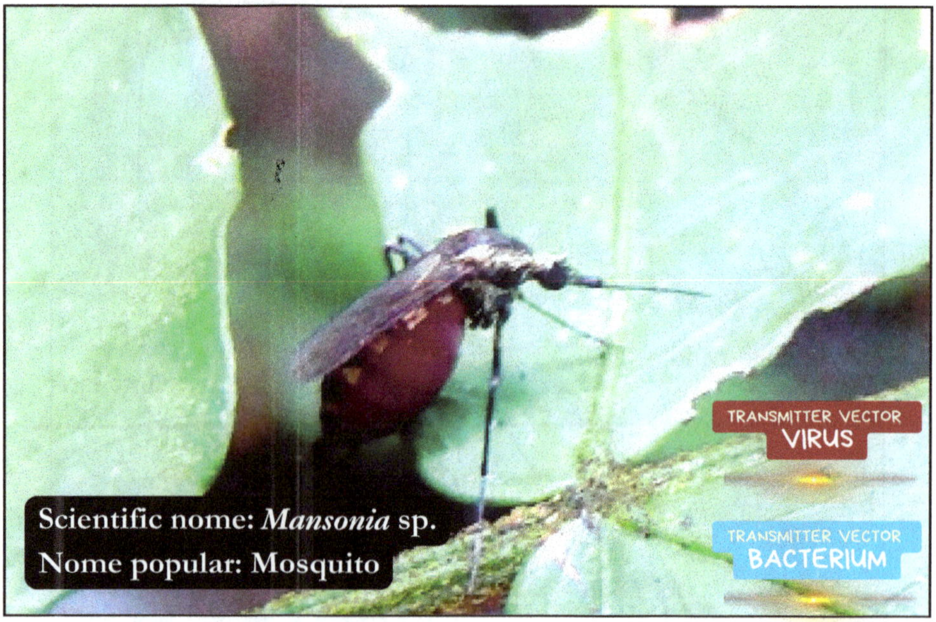

In the images above, two female mosquitoes are shown fully engorged with blood — unfortunately, drawn from the author during his expeditions through the Amazon rainforest. However, since this is an endemic area for yellow fever, his vaccination is up to date. For now, he remains protected from the main disease these mosquitoes could transmit to him.

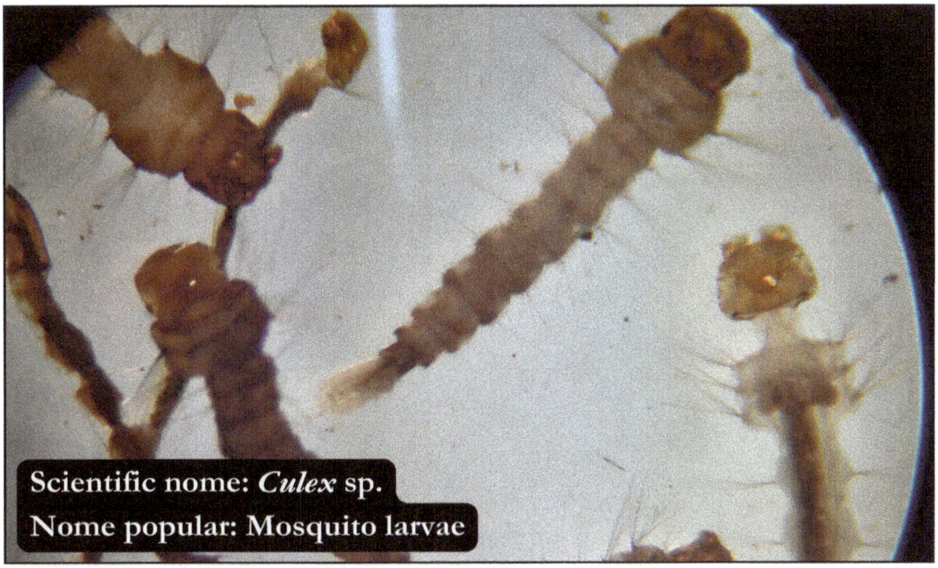

Part of the mosquito life cycle takes place in water. Here we see developing larvae feeding on organic debris and sediments. Soon, they will transform into pupae and undergo metamorphosis until they reach the adult flying stage.

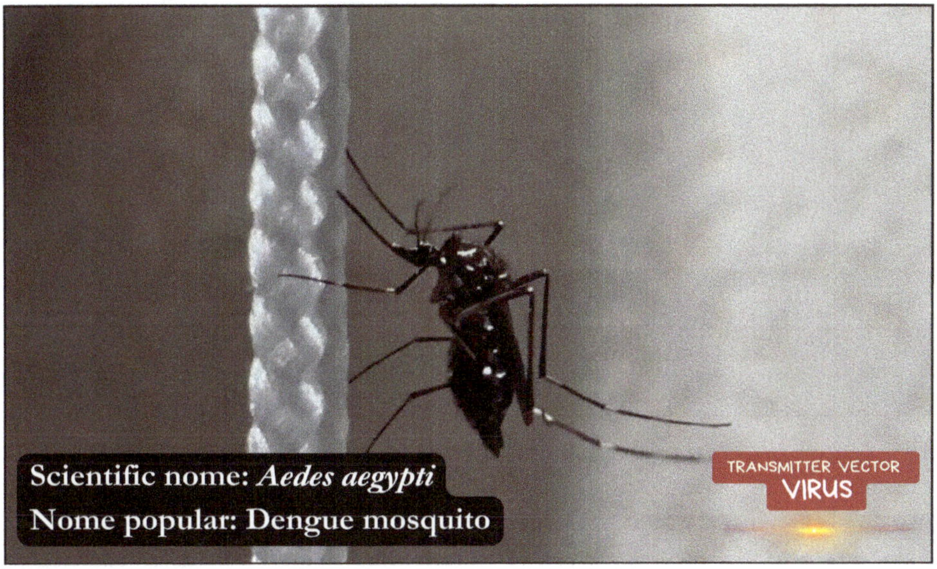

Now in their winged (flying) stage, female mosquitoes begin searching for a blood meal, while males typically feed on nectar and sugary substances to gain energy for flying and finding mates. Their antennae are sensory tools, capable of detecting the carbon dioxide (CO_2) we exhale, helping them locate potential hosts.

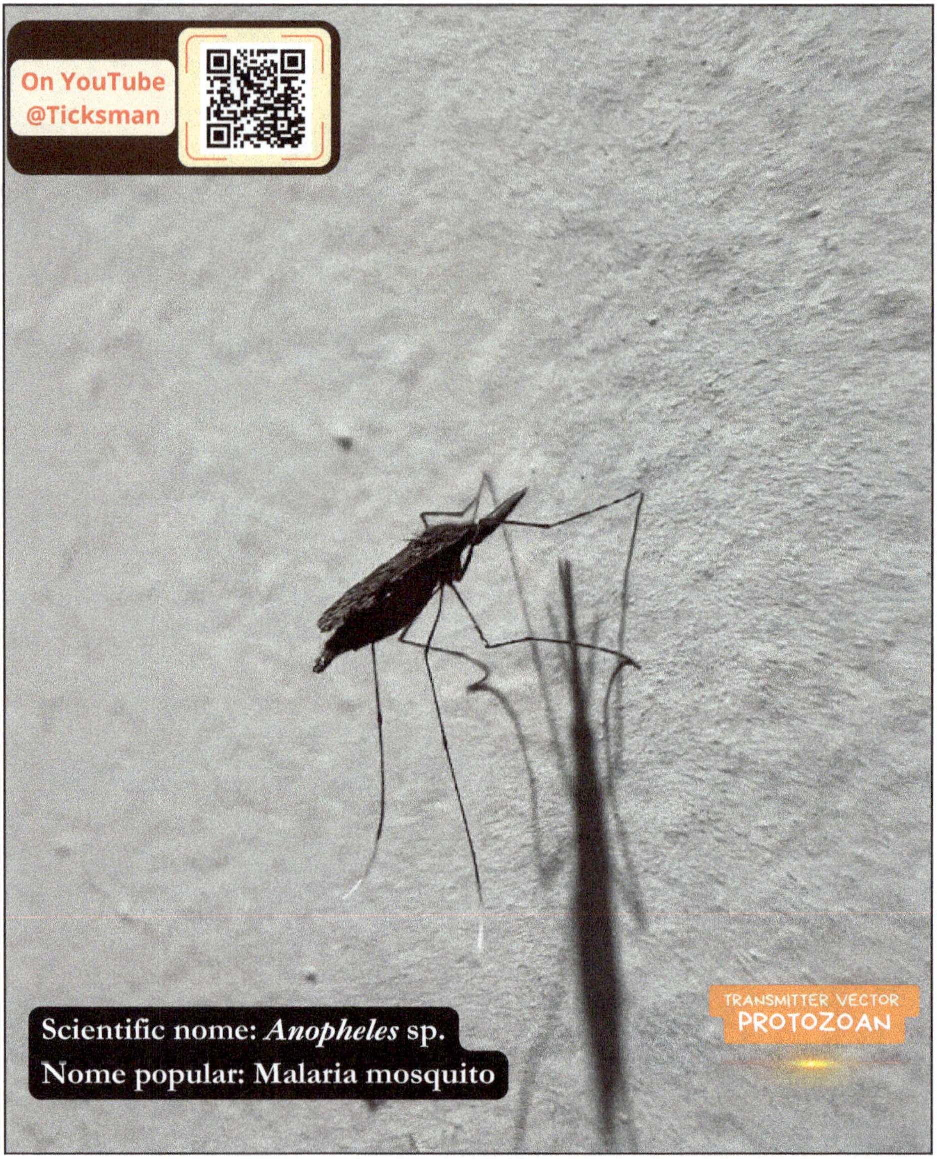
On YouTube
@Ticksman
Scientific nome: Anopheles sp.
Nome popular: Malaria mosquito
TRANSMITTER VECTOR
PROTOZOAN

The *Anopheles* mosquito is one of the most feared in the world—especially in Africa, the Americas, and Asia—because it transmits malaria, causing millions of new cases each year and over 750,000 deaths. This mosquito adapts well to a variety of environments and thrives near humans… or maybe it's humans who choose to live near them? Either way, always use repellents and avoid being outdoors during peak biting hours—between 5–7 AM and 5–8 PM in endemic areas. That way, you reduce your risk of being bitten by infected females and contracting malaria. If you develop symptoms after visiting a risk area, seek medical attention immediately—early diagnosis means a high chance of cure.

Fleas: Tiny Jumping Vampires in Your Home

They are small, fast, and jump like acrobats. You might not even notice them… until the itching starts.

Fleas are one of the most common parasites found in homes—especially where dogs and cats live. They're not just annoying; they can also transmit dangerous diseases to both animals and humans.

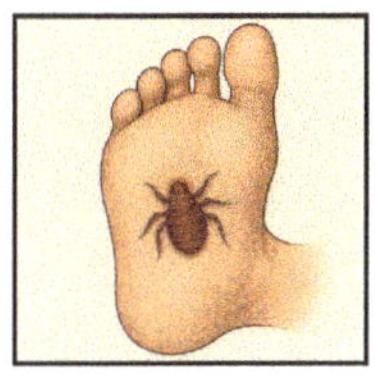

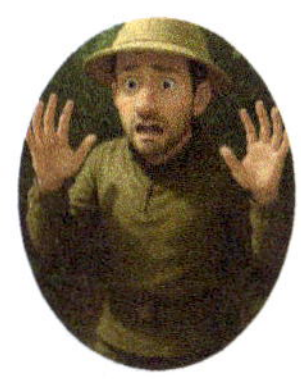

Why Should You Care?

Fleas can transmit:

- Tapeworms (*Dipylidium caninum*) — to pets and sometimes to children.
- Cat Scratch Disease — indirectly, by infecting cats with *Bartonella henselae.*
- Flea Allergy Dermatitis — causing intense itching and inflammation.
- And most historically... the **Black Death** (Bubonic Plague).

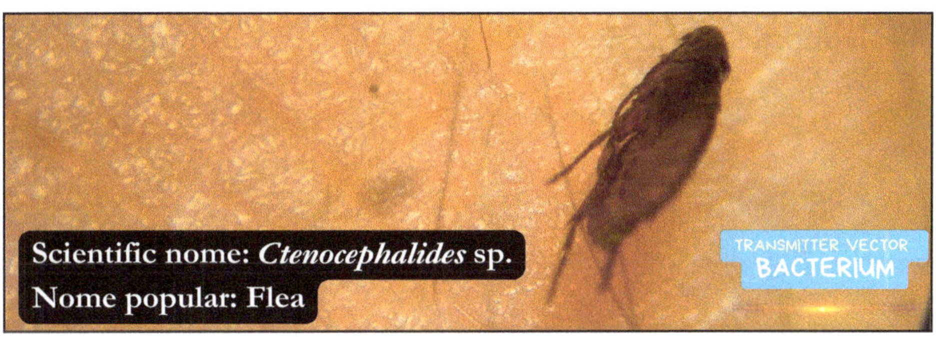
Scientific nome: Ctenocephalides sp.
Nome popular: Flea
TRANSMITTER VECTOR
BACTERIUM

Dog fleas can be extremely bloodthirsty, and in many cases, they may bite humans when the infestation on the pet is severe. That's why it's essential to take your pet to the veterinarian regularly for proper care and parasite prevention.

The Black Death: When Fleas Changed History

In the 14th century, a tiny flea helped unleash the deadliest pandemic in human history — the **Black Death**, which killed more than 75 million people in Europe, Asia, and Africa.

How did it happen?

1. Fleas infested infected rodents, carrying the bacterium *Yersinia pestis.*
2. Inside the flea, the bacteria multiplied rapidly, clogging the flea's mouthpart.
3. The flea, unable to feed properly, became desperately hungry, biting again and again.
4. Every time it bit, it regurgitated infected saliva, spreading the plague to new hosts—animals and humans alike.

There are three types of plague:

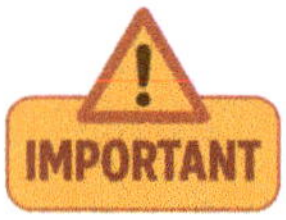

- **Bubonic** – causes swollen lymph nodes (buboes); most common.

- **Pneumonic** – affects the lungs; highly contagious via droplets.

- **Septicemic** – spreads in the bloodstream; can cause death in hours if untreated.

Flea Life Cycle: The Hidden Threat

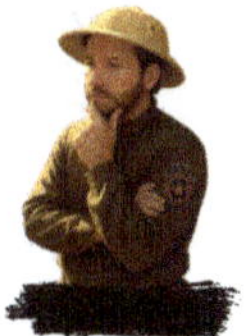

Fleas go through four life stages:

1. **Eggs** – laid on pets but fall into carpets, furniture, and floor cracks.
2. **Larvae** – feed on organic material and flea dirt (adult feces).
3. **Pupae** – develop in cocoons; can wait weeks to months to emerge.
4. **Adults** – jump onto hosts, feed on blood, and reproduce.

One female flea can lay up to 50 eggs per day!

How to Eliminate Fleas: Total Protection Plan

1. Treat All Pets Regularly

- Use vet-approved flea control: oral, topical, or flea collars.

2. Vacuum Daily During Infestations

- Focus on carpets, pet beds, sofas, and corners.
- Immediately discard the vacuum bag outside the home.

3. Wash Everything

- Wash pet bedding, blankets, and soft toys in hot water weekly.

4. Avoid Carpets

- Carpets are ideal flea egg incubators. Use rugs or washable mats in pet areas.

5. Use Outdoor Water Smartly

- Recycle soapy water from laundry to flood flea-prone areas in the yard.
- Flea eggs don't hatch well in very moist or soapy conditions.

6. Spray and Fog Responsibly

- Use insect growth regulators (IGRs) and safe flea sprays indoors and in pet zones.

7. Don't Forget the Yard

- Fleas love shady spots and dog houses. Keep lawns trimmed and clean.

Curious Case: The "Bicho-de-pé" (*Tunga penetrans*)

Meet the tiniest flea with the biggest impact — *Tunga penetrans*, also known as the chigoe flea or jigger, famous in parts of Latin America and Africa.

- It burrows into bare feet, especially around toenails or soles.
- Once inside, it grows rapidly, feeding on your blood and laying eggs from under your skin.
- It causes pain, swelling, and in some cases, serious secondary infections.

Prevention tips:

- Always wear shoes, even in sandy or rural areas.
- Avoid walking barefoot in places with animal droppings or loose soil.
- If you suspect you've been infected, don't try to remove it at home—go to a hospital or clinic to prevent complications.

Fun Fact

Fleas can jump up to 33 cm (13 in) vertically—more than 100 times their body length. If you could jump like that, you'd leap over a building!

Final Note for Parasite Hunters

Fleas may be tiny, but their impact can be enormous.

With smart cleaning, consistent treatment, and a bit of science, you can defend your home and protect your pets—and yourself—from these persistent parasites.

Stay alert, stay informed, and remember:

Knowledge is the best repellant!

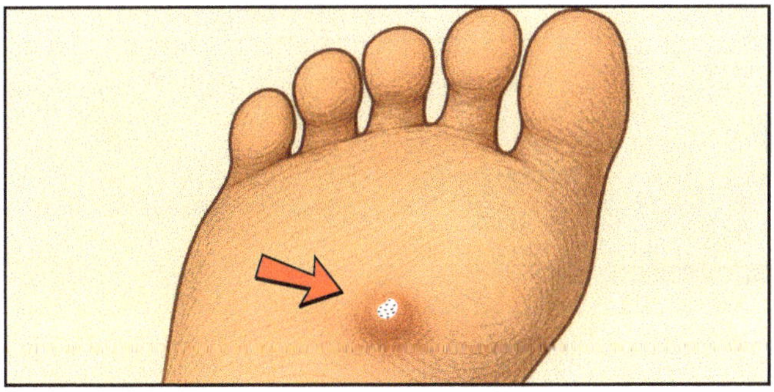

If you find a jigger (*Tunga penetrans*) on your dog, cat, pig, or another pet, be careful—these fleas won't hesitate to try your skin too. Protect your animals, and you'll be protecting yourself too!

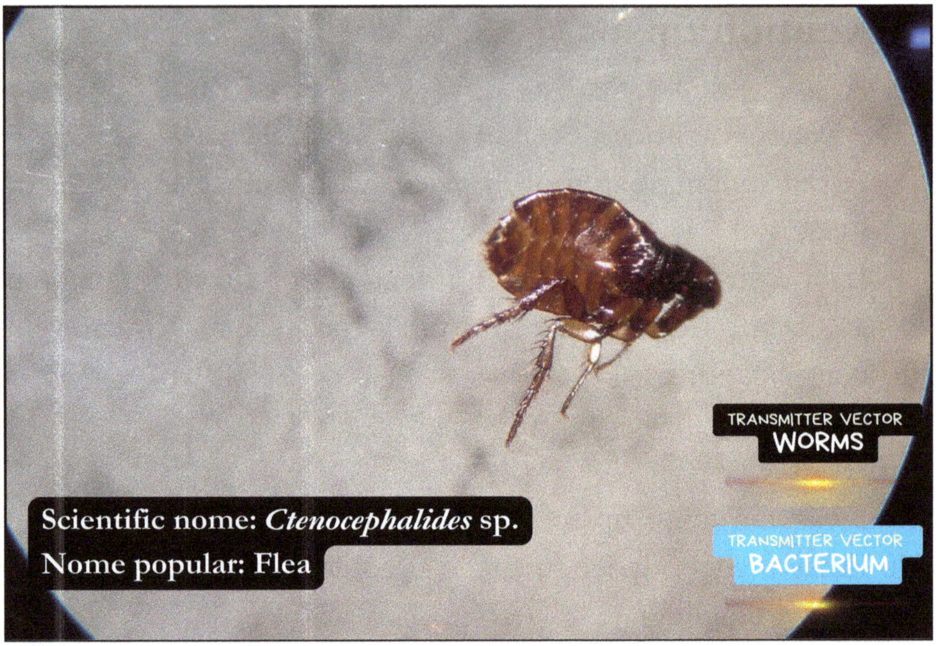
TRANSMITTER VECTOR
WORMS
Scientific nome: Ctenocephalides sp.
Nome popular: Flea
TRANSMITTER VECTOR
BACTERIUM

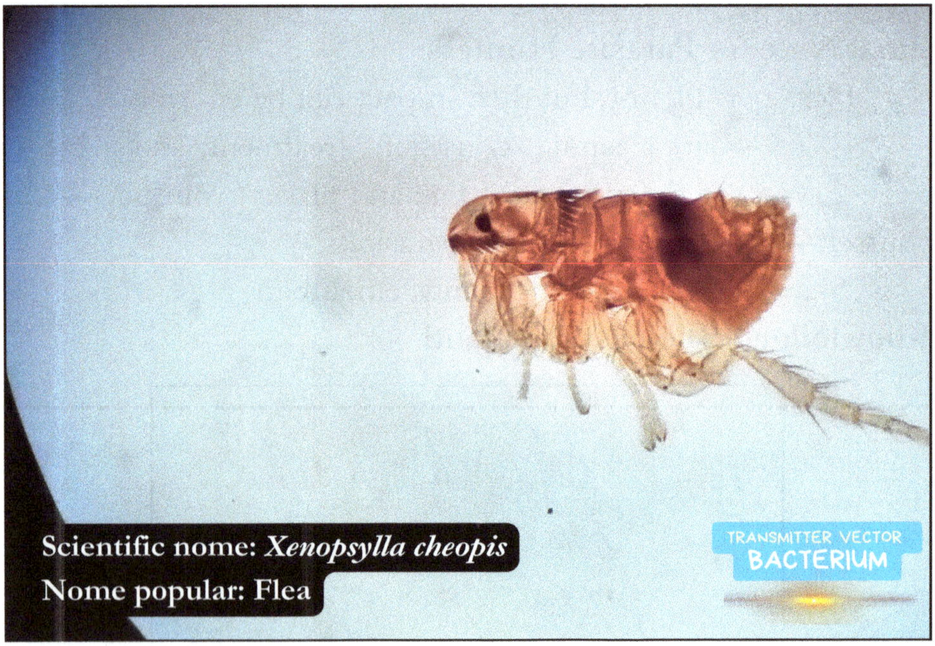
Scientific nome: Xenopsylla cheopis
Nome popular: Flea
TRANSMITTER VECTOR
BACTERIUM

Black Death flea observed under the microscope. This ectoparasite is laterally flattened, allowing it to move easily between hairs and narrow crevices on its host. It is covered in sensory bristles and equipped with powerful hind legs, enabling it to jump great distances relative to its size. Fleas played a major role in the spread of the plague by transmitting *Yersinia pestis* bacteria between rodents and humans.

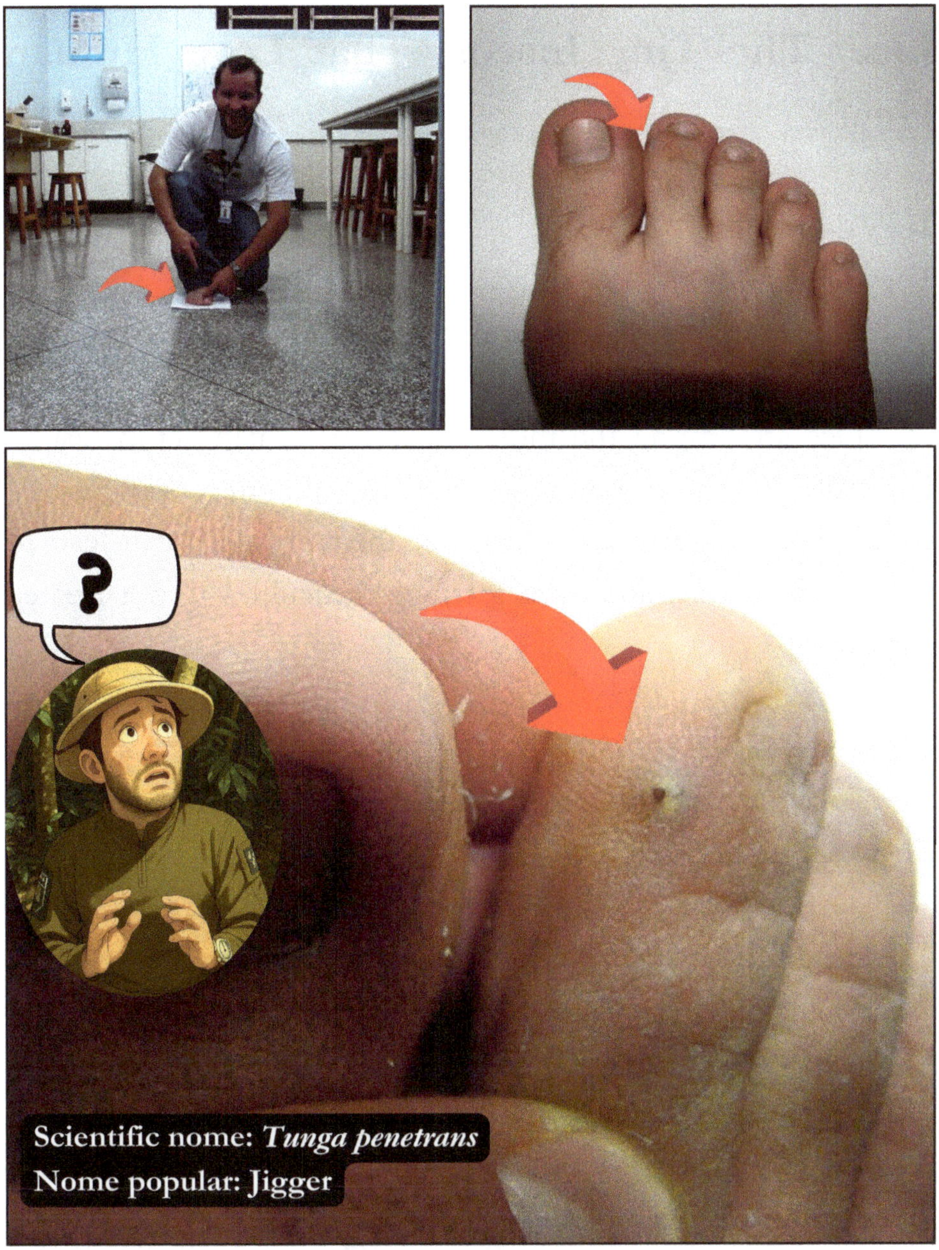

*Tunga penetran*s, commonly known as the chigoe flea or 'jigger', penetrates the skin—not only on the feet, but also on other body parts. Once embedded, the female feeds and swells in size as she develops eggs. In some cultures, extraction is performed mechanically using a needle, but without proper asepsis, this can lead to secondary infections. When in doubt, seek medical attention, as multiple infestations can occur across the body.

Lice: The Tiny Insects That Love Human Heads

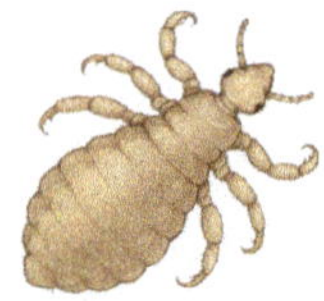

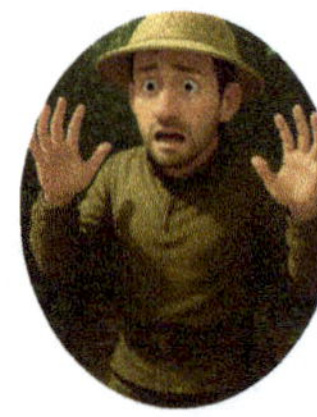

They don't jump.
They don't fly.

But they crawl—fast and cling tightly to hair like expert gymnasts.

Lice are among the most persistent human ectoparasites, especially common among school-age children around the world. These insects are small, but their presence can lead to itching, infections, and even learning difficulties if not treated correctly.

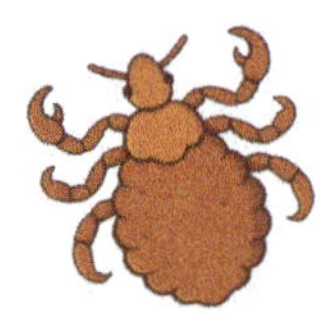

What Are Lice?

Lice are wingless insects that live exclusively on humans. There are three types:

1. Head Louse (*Pediculus humanus capitis*)
   - Found on the scalp and hair, especially near the ears and nape of the neck.
2. Body Louse (*Pediculus humanus humanus*)
   - Lives in clothing seams, moving to the skin to feed. More common in overcrowded or unhygienic conditions.
3. Pubic Louse (*Pthirus pubis*), also called "crab louse" or "crabs"
   - Infests pubic hair, but may also be found in armpits, chest hair, eyebrows, or eyelashes.

The Life Cycle: Fast and Sticky

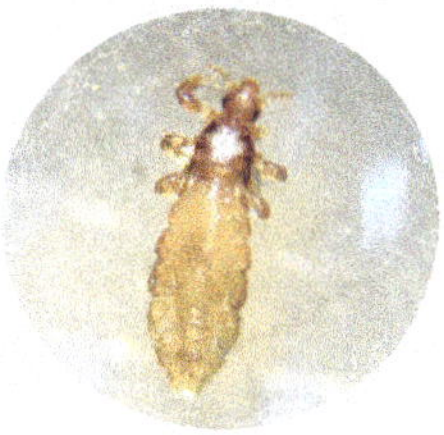

Lice go through three stages:

1. **Nit (Egg)** – Tiny, white or yellowish, and glued to hair strands near the scalp.
    - A single female can lay up to 10 eggs per day, totaling more than 100 eggs in her lifetime!
    - Nits hatch in 7–10 days.
2. **Nymph** – Young lice that mature into adults in about 10 days.
3. **Adult Louse** – About 2–3 mm long, they feed on blood several times a day.

Important Note:

The white specks you see on the hair? Those are nits—and they don't fall off easily, which is why they need to be combed or manually removed.

What Can Lice Cause?

- Itching from saliva injected during feeding.
- Pediculosis – A skin condition caused by excessive lice, leading to sores, bleeding, and bacterial infections.
- Sleep disturbances and irritability.
- In children, studies show up to 40% may experience attention and focus difficulties due to constant itching and discomfort.

Though lice are not always associated with disease, body lice can transmit:

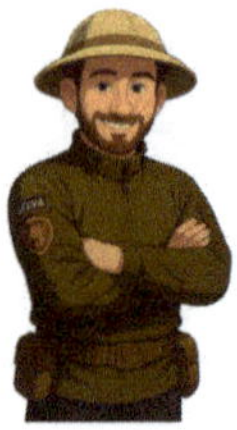

- Typhus (*Rickettsia prowazekii*)
- Relapsing fever (*Borrelia recurrentis*)
- Trench fever (*Bartonella quintana*)

These diseases are serious and were devastating during wars and in refugee camps.

How to Get Rid of Lice: Battle Plan

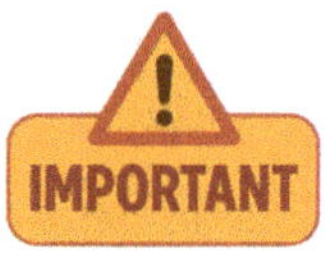

1. Use Lice Treatments

- Over-the-counter pediculicides like permethrin or pyrethrin.
- Prescription shampoos (e.g., malathion, ivermectin) in stubborn cases.

2. Manual Nit Removal

- Use a fine-toothed metal lice comb daily for at least 10–14 days.
- Divide the hair into small sections and check thoroughly.

3. Wash and Disinfect

- Wash bedding, clothing, hats, and hair accessories in hot water (60°C / 140°F) and dry on high heat.
- Seal unwashable items in a plastic bag for 2 weeks.

4. Vacuum Your Home

- Vacuum pillows, couches, car seats, and anywhere the head or body may have rested.

5. Check and Treat Contacts

- All household members should be checked and treated if infested.

Fun Fact

Lice have existed for millions of years, and each species is specialized to live only on humans.

They can survive up to 36 hours off the body, which is why it's crucial to treat both the person and their environment.

A Note for Families and Teachers

Head lice don't mean someone is "dirty." They spread through direct head-to-head contact, which is common during play, hugs, or selfies.

Avoiding panic, treating early, and staying informed is the best way to keep schools, families, and communities lice-free. Let's keep heads happy—and itch-free!

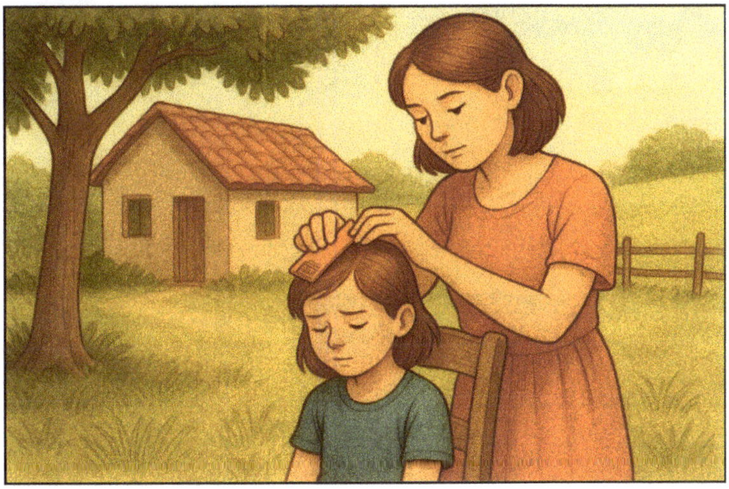

A mother carefully inspects her daughter's hair using a fine-tooth comb—known in Brazil as "pente fino"—to remove lice eggs (nits) and adult lice. It's common during this process for mothers to squeeze and crush the lice between their fingernails to kill them.

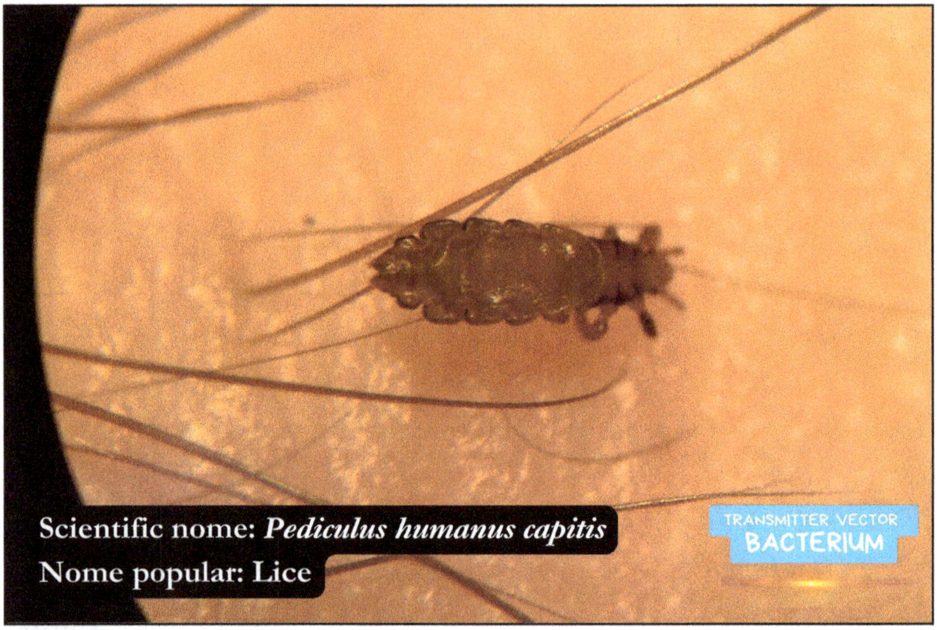

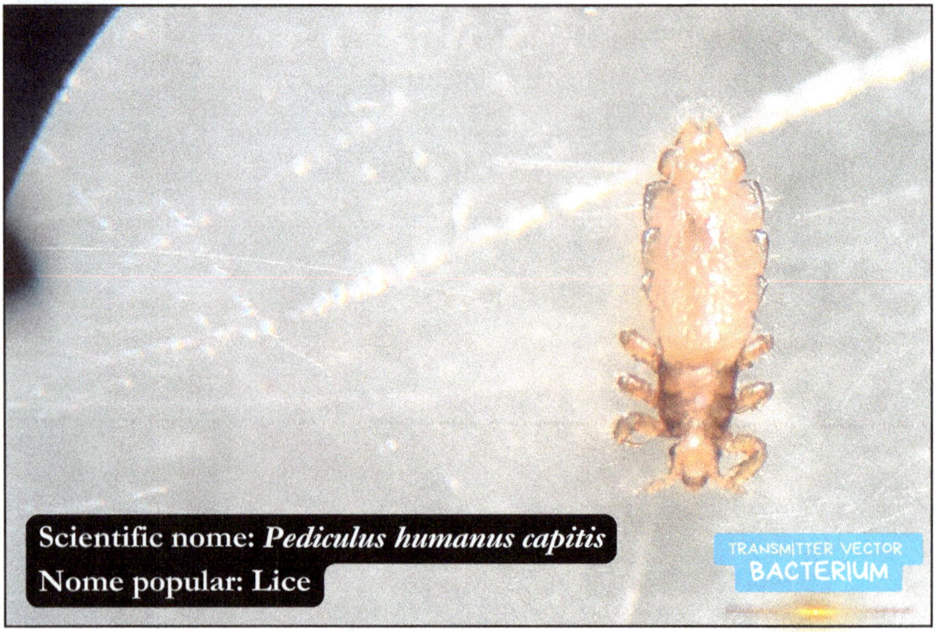

Head lice (*Pediculus humanus capitis*) are wingless and cannot jump, but they are well adapted for clinging to hair with their clawed legs. In schools, close contact—such as hugging or sharing fabric-covered chairs—can easily spread lice from one child to another. A louse may crawl onto a chair and remain hidden, waiting for the next host to sit down. Regular checks and hygiene measures are key to preventing infestations.

The Night Is Not Always Safe: The Bed Bug Invasion

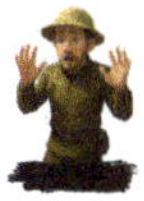

Imagine this: You're fast asleep, dreaming of adventures in the Amazon rainforest... and somewhere, hidden in the folds of your pillow, a tiny army of vampires is on the move.

- They don't fly.
- They don't live on your pet.
- They don't even carry diseases like ticks or mosquitoes.

But they feed on your blood, and they're some of the hardest insects to eliminate once they've moved in.
Welcome to the surreal world of bed bugs.

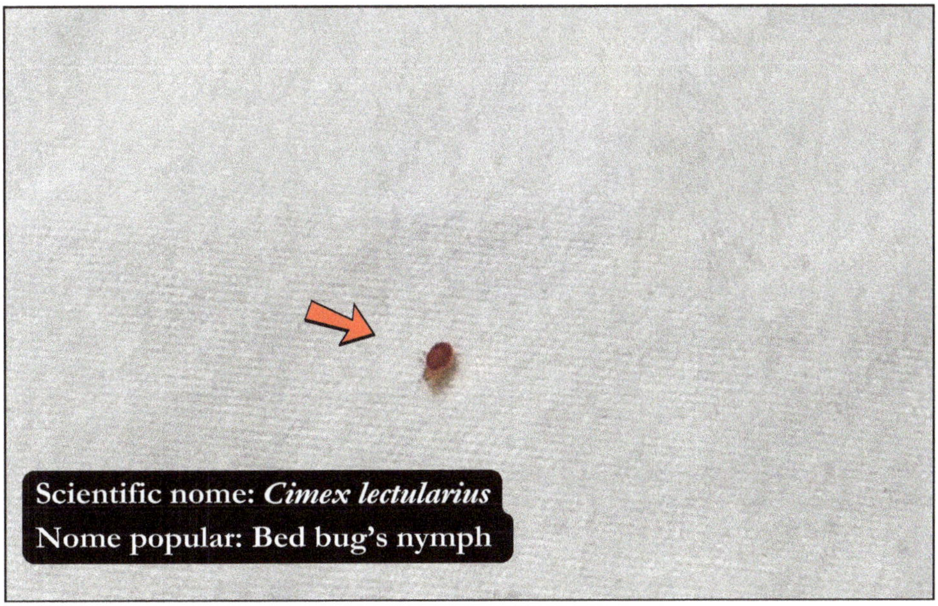

Here we see an immature stage of a bed bug, visibly engorged with the author's blood during a trip to the United States in 2019. Infestations in mattresses from hotels, cruise ships, and homes are common worldwide. Bed bugs are stealthy nocturnal feeders, often hiding in crevices and seams during the day—making regular inspection and cleanliness essential to avoid bites and spread.

Why Should You Care?

While bed bugs are not known to transmit diseases, they can cause:

- Intense allergic skin reactions (itchy red welts, blisters)
- Sleep disorders and anxiety
- Secondary infections from scratching
- Social and psychological stress, especially in children

They've become a public health nuisance in homes, hotels, dormitories, and even airplanes—in the US, Europe, and nearly every continent (yes, even Antarctica has monitoring protocols!).

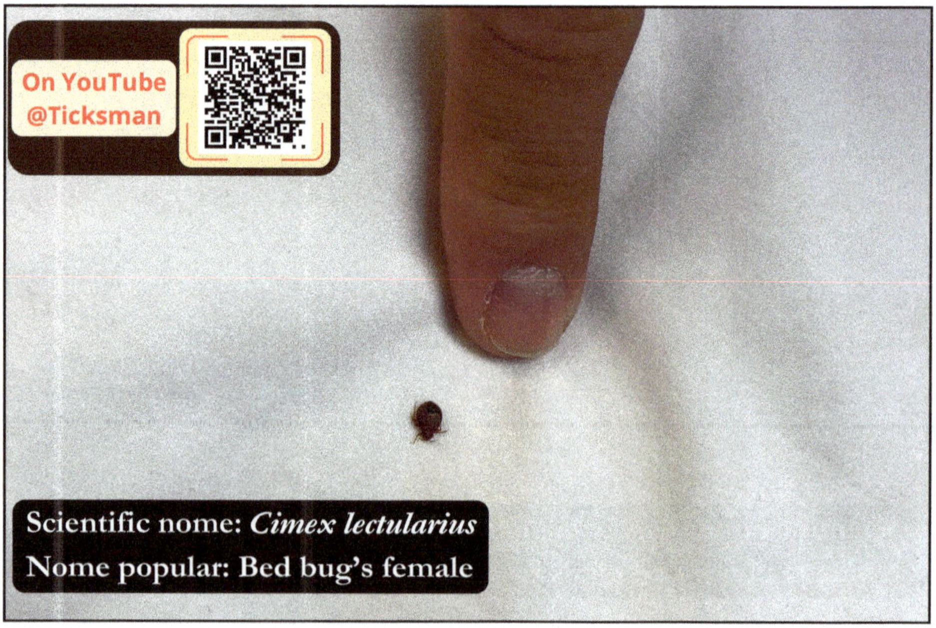

This image shows a large female bed bug found attempting to bite the author's neck at 2 a.m. Sensing something unusual, he woke up, turned on the light—and there she was, hungry. Now imagine how many people are bitten each night without even knowing that a whole family of bloodthirsty insects might be living right under their sheets. Bed bugs are expert hiders and silent feeders—awareness is your first line of defense.

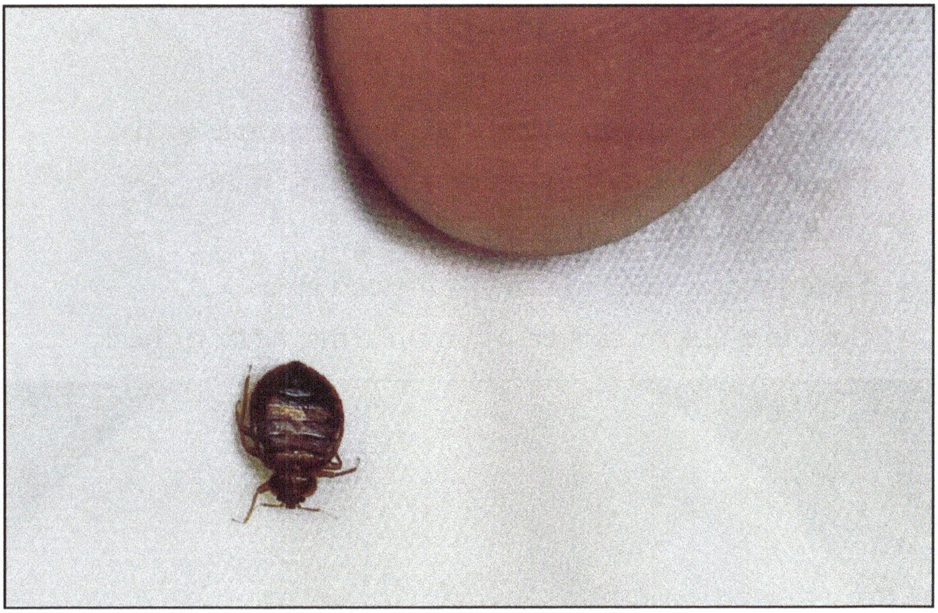

Female bedbug found in a hotel bed during a trip. It is very common in these places to have carpets and rugs on the floor to avoid noise from suitcases and people walking, but this is ideal for the proliferation of this insect.

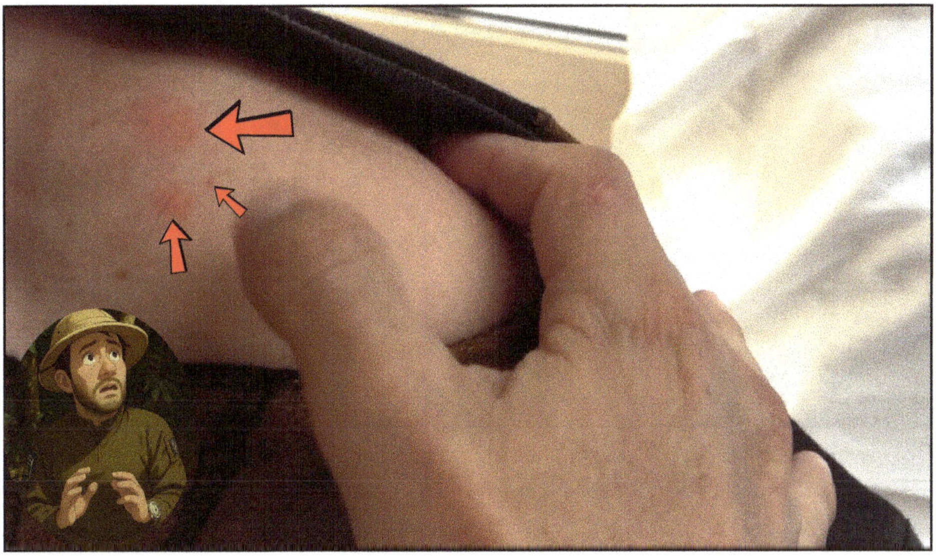

Injury to the author's shoulder caused by multiple bites from bed bug nymphs and adults. Also documented in a video for Youtube in Portuguese.

How to Spot a Bed Bug Invasion

- Tiny reddish-brown insects, shaped like apple seeds
- Blood stains or dark spots on sheets and mattresses
- Shed exoskeletons (they molt!)
- Sweet, musty odor in heavily infested areas
- Bites in a line or cluster, often on arms, neck, or back

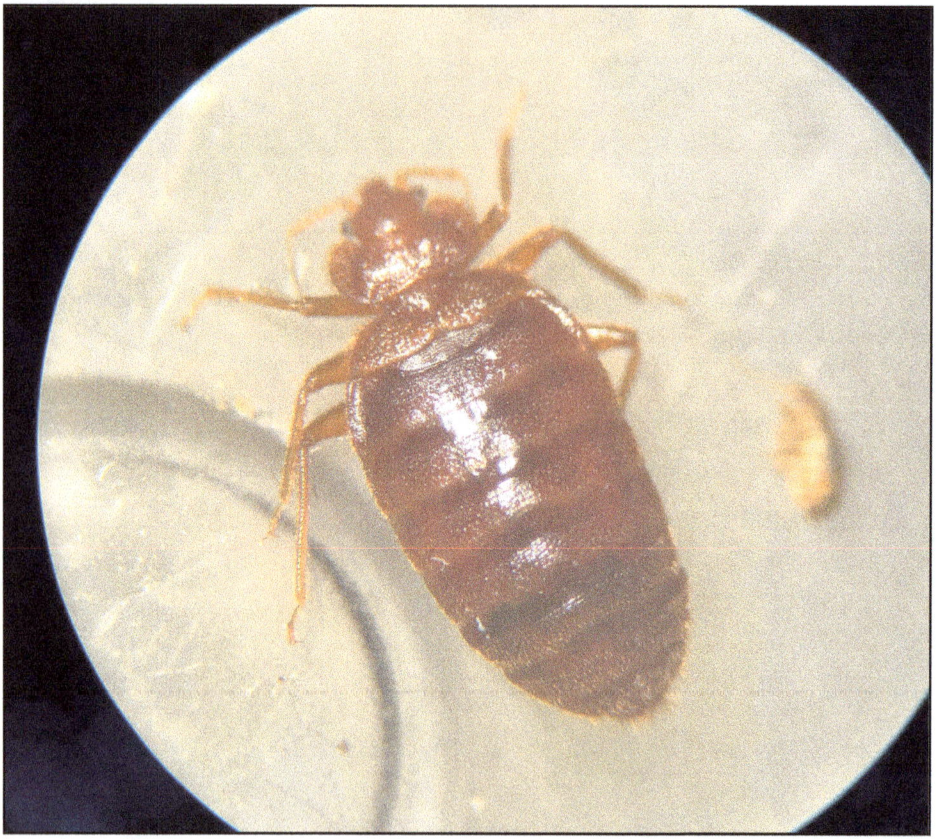

Bed bug observed under a stereoscopic magnifier in a laboratory for scientific identification. Note its distinct reddish-brown color, enlarged abdomen filled with blood, and clearly visible morphological features such as the segmented antennae, prominent compound eyes, and six legs adapted for crawling. These characteristics are key for identifying bed bugs, especially in early infestation stages. Their flat, oval-shaped bodies allow them to hide in narrow cracks and seams of mattresses, furniture, and walls—making them elusive but not invisible to the trained eye.

Your Bed Bug Battle Plan: The Ultimate Guide

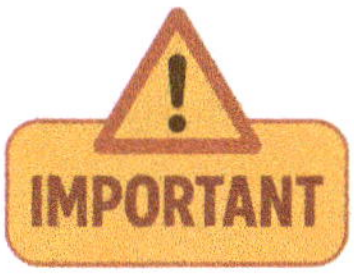

1. Declutter & Detect

- Strip beds completely.
- Use a flashlight and a credit card to search seams, mattress edges, behind headboards, under nightstands.
- Use interceptors under bed legs to trap them.

2. Vacuum Like a Warrior

- Vacuum everything: mattresses, box springs, carpets, bed frames, and even electrical outlets!
- Immediately seal the vacuum bag in plastic and dispose of it outside.

3. Wash & Roast Them

- Wash bedding, clothes, stuffed animals on high heat.
- Dry for at least 30 minutes on the highest dryer setting—heat kills all life stages.

4. Isolate & Protect

- Encase mattresses and pillows with bed bug-proof covers (zipped and sealed).
- Pull beds away from walls, and don't let blankets touch the floor.

5. Freeze the Sneaky Survivors

- Place small infested items in a sealed bag in the freezer at −18°C (0°F) for at least 4 days.

6. Chemical Defense

- Use only bed bug-specific insecticides (pyrethroids, desiccants).
- Be cautious: bed bugs in many regions have developed resistance.
- Always consult pest control experts for heavy infestations.

7. Steam Like a Pro

- A powerful steam cleaner with temperatures above 60°C (140°F) can penetrate fabrics and crevices—instantly lethal to bed bugs.

8. Repeat the Cycle

- Eggs may hatch days later—repeat cleaning and inspections every 7–10 days for at least a month.

Important Note:
Hire a specialized pest control company or consult a professional. Many insecticides and pest control products can be harmful to humans and domestic animals like dogs and cats. Don't take unnecessary risks—do it right and stay safe. Protect your health and your home.

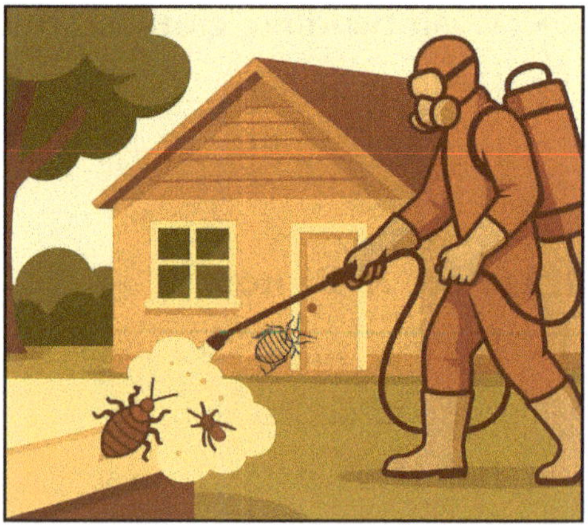

Fun Fact: Bed Bugs Are Ancient

Fossils show that bed bugs have been feeding on humans for over 3,500 years. That's right—they've adapted to us since the time of the Pharaohs.

The Magic of Prevention

- Don't bring secondhand furniture inside without inspecting it thoroughly.
- After hotel stays, leave luggage outside and heat-treat clothes immediately.
- Use protective covers and bed barriers at home.

Final Word for the Brave Parasite Hunters:

Bed bugs don't jump or fly. They crawl. And when you know where they crawl… you can win the war.

So grab your flashlight, sharpen your instincts, and remember—even the tiniest creatures can be defeated with knowledge and consistency.

Let's keep our nights peaceful—and our sheets bug-free.

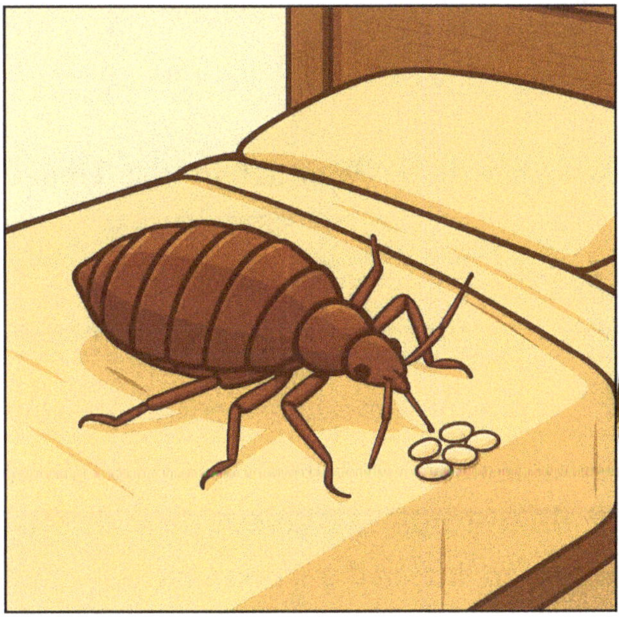

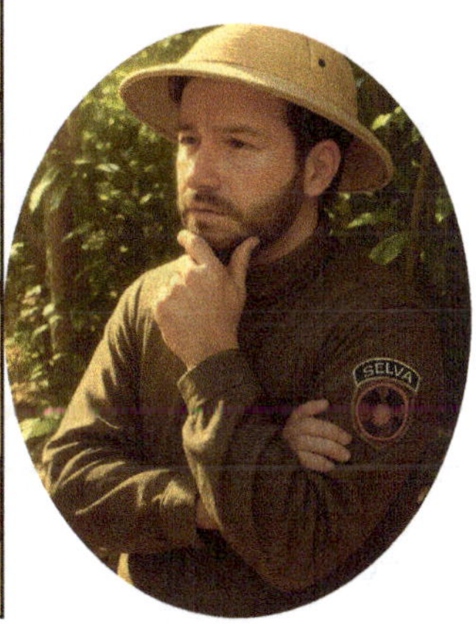

Assassin Bugs (Kissing Bugs): The Silent Messengers of Chagas Disease

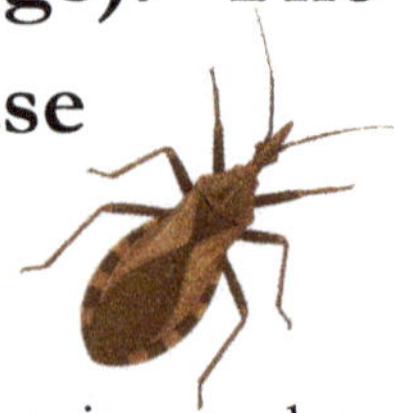

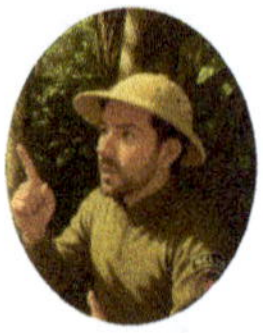

They don't roar. They don't buzz.

They move quietly at night, hiding in cracks and straw roofs.

They wait, patient and silent—then come out to feed… not just on blood, but on a life-changing parasite.

Welcome to the world of the "assassin bug", known scientifically as the Triatomine bug, and feared for spreading one of the most underestimated diseases of our time: Chagas disease (American Trypanosomiasis).

Where in the World?

There are more than 170 species of Triatomine bugs, mostly found in Central and South America, but the disease is no longer limited to tropical areas.

Today (2025):

- Over 400,000 cases have been reported in the United States.
- More than 80,000 people are infected in Europe.
- Thousands of cases have emerged in Japan and other parts of Asia.

Many of these infections occurred through blood transfusions, when the disease was not screened in donors, especially immigrants who were infected unknowingly.

The Life Cycle of the Assassin Bug

1. **Egg** – Laid in cracks or near sleeping areas.
2. **Nymph** – Passes through five stages, feeding on blood at each.
3. **Adult** – Fully winged, active at night, and lives in dark, warm hiding spots.

They feed by piercing the skin with their mouthparts—but that's not how they transmit the parasite.

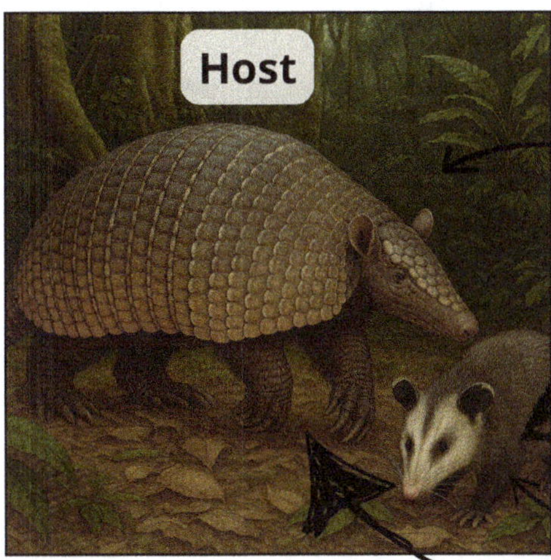

For each stage it is necessary to feed on the blood of some animal, and if this animal is contaminated with the protozoan, the insect becomes contaminated.

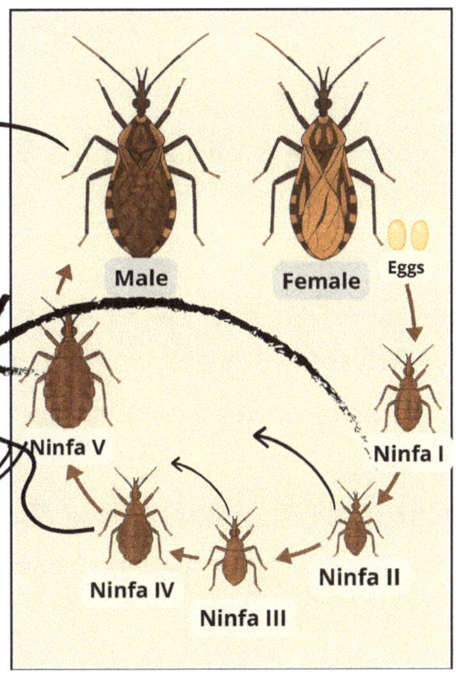

How Chagas Disease Is Transmitted

Chagas is caused by the protozoan *Trypanosoma cruzi*, and the main form of transmission is not through the bite, but through infected feces left near the wound, eyes, or mouth after the insect feeds.

Other transmission methods:

- Mother-to-child during pregnancy (congenital transmission).
- Contaminated blood transfusions or organ transplants.
- Laboratory accidents.
- Consumption of contaminated food or drink (like sugarcane juice or açaí in the Amazon).
- If Triatomine bugs fall into the grinder, especially when lights are placed above food-processing areas, they may be crushed along with the fruit, leading to oral infection.

Signs and Symptoms

Acute Chagas Disease (First Weeks)

- Fever
- Fatigue
- Swelling near the eye or bite site (Romaña's sign)
- Rash, headache, or swollen lymph nodes

Symptoms often go unnoticed or are confused with common illnesses.

Chronic Chagas Disease (Years Later)

- May be asymptomatic for decades
- Can progress to:
    - Heart disease (arrhythmias, heart failure, sudden death)
    - Digestive system disorders (enlarged esophagus or colon)
    - Neurological complications

Once in the chronic stage, there is no definitive cure—which makes early diagnosis crucial.

How to Prevent Chagas Disease

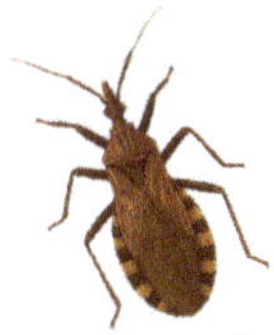

1. Avoid the Bug

- Seal cracks in walls, roofs, and window frames—especially in rural homes.
- Use mosquito nets and insect screens, especially at night.
- Keep domestic animals outdoors, as they can attract Triatomines.

2. Process Açaí and Sugarcane Safely

- NEVER install lights above grinding machines—they attract bugs.
- Wash all fruits thoroughly.
- Use closed facilities with proper food safety protocols.

3. Be Aware of Blood and Organ Transfusions

- In non-endemic countries, ensure blood donors are screened for Chagas.
- Medical professionals must be trained in detection and prevention.

4. Monitor Pregnant Women from Endemic Regions

- Screen for *T. cruzi* during prenatal care to prevent congenital transmission.

5. Seek Medical Care Immediately

- If you notice suspicious symptoms or suspect exposure, consult a doctor quickly.
- Early diagnosis = best chance for treatment.

Fun Fact

Chagas disease was discovered by Brazilian physician Carlos Chagas in 1909. He was the first to describe the parasite, vector, host, and disease—all in one study. A true hero of tropical medicine!

Final Thought for Brave Parasite Hunters

The assassin bug doesn't just strike in the jungle—it may be hidden in food, in houses, or even in blood bags.

But with knowledge, sanitation, and early diagnosis, we can stop the silent spread of this tropical intruder.

Let's protect our families, our food, and our futures—Chagas disease is preventable.

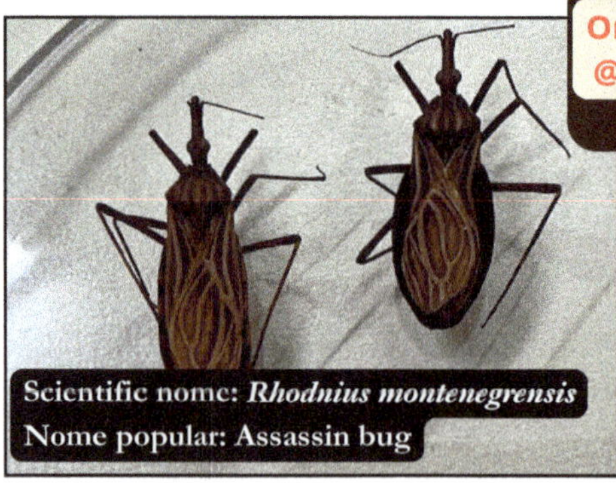

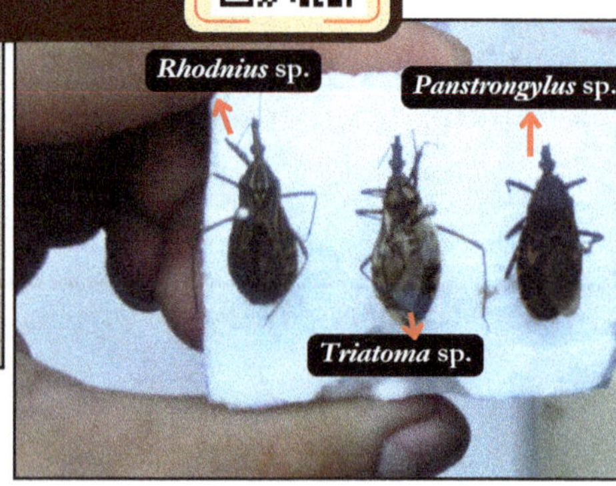

Photo at top: Here we see two assassin bugs (kissing bugs), notorious vectors of Chagas disease, commonly found across South America. Photo below: The three most prevalent genera—*Rhodnius, Triatoma,* and *Panstrongylus*—inhabit a variety of environments such as forested areas, tree trunks, animal burrows, bat caves, chicken coops, pigsties, cattle pens, and even inside homes. If you spot one of these insects, follow your local Health Ministry's guidelines immediately. When it comes to Chagas disease, caution is never too much.

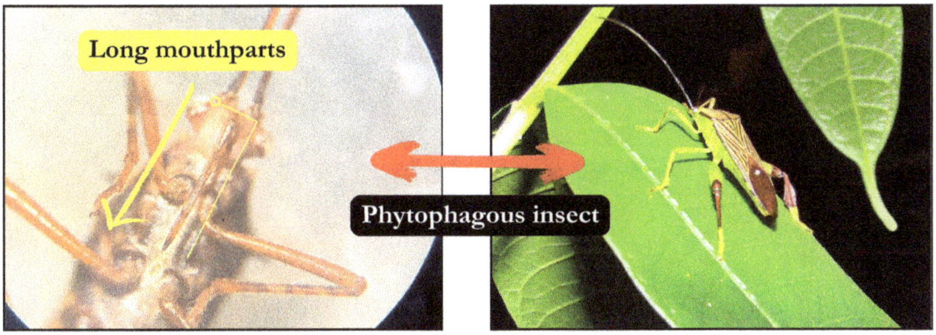

True bugs can be classified by their feeding habits based on the structure of their mouthparts. **(1)** Phytophagous bugs feed on plant sap, with a long proboscis extending beyond the first pair of legs.

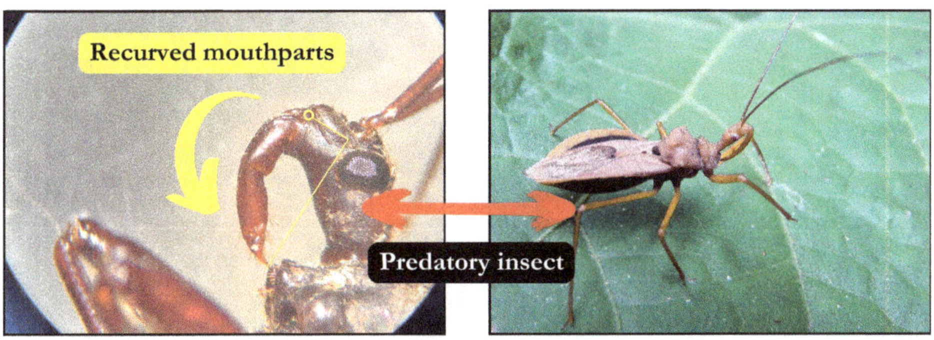

(2) Predatory bugs feed on other insects and have a shorter, robust mouthpart—though their bite is painful, they do not transmit diseases.

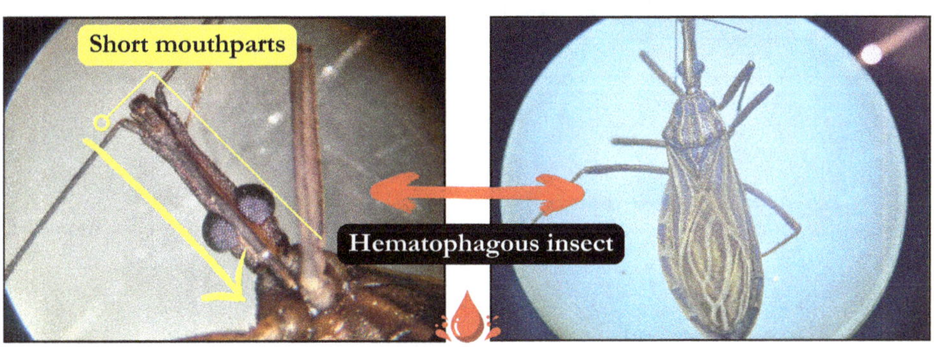

(3) Hematophagous bugs, such as kissing bugs, feed on blood, with a proboscis that does not extend past the first leg pair, and they can transmit serious diseases like Chagas

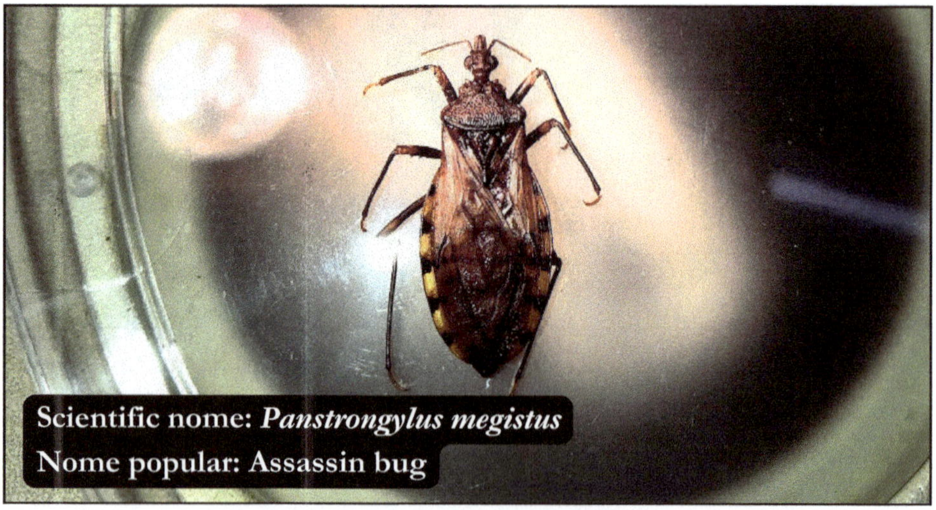
Scientific nome: *Panstrongylus megistus*
Nome popular: Assassin bug

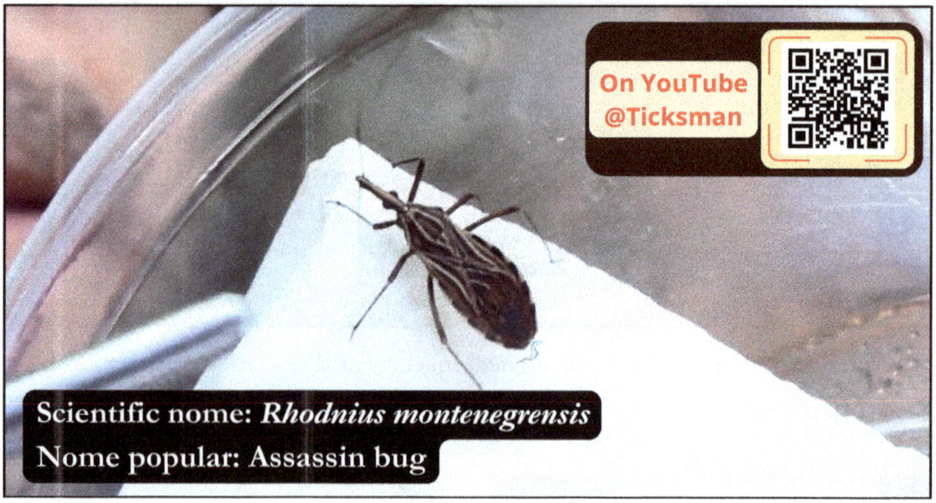
On YouTube
@Ticksman
Scientific nome: *Rhodnius montenegrensis*
Nome popular: Assassin bug

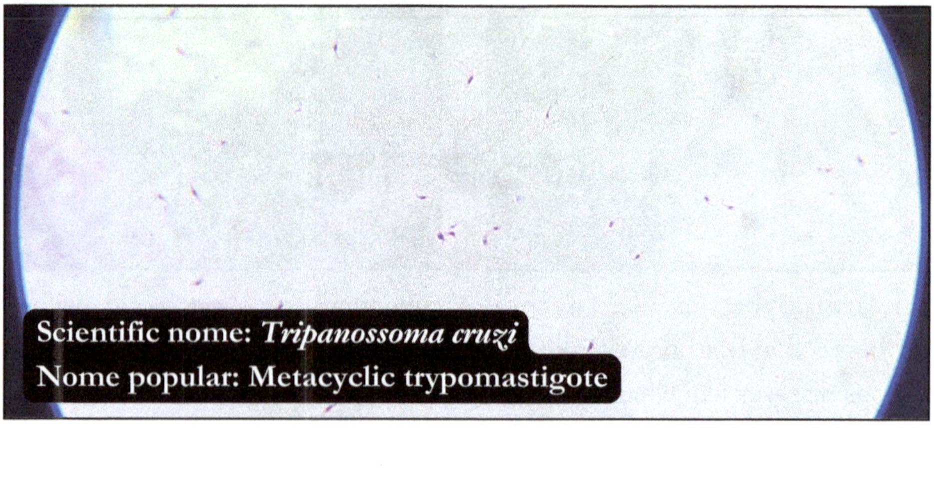
Scientific nome: *Tripanossoma cruzi*
Nome popular: Metacyclic trypomastigote

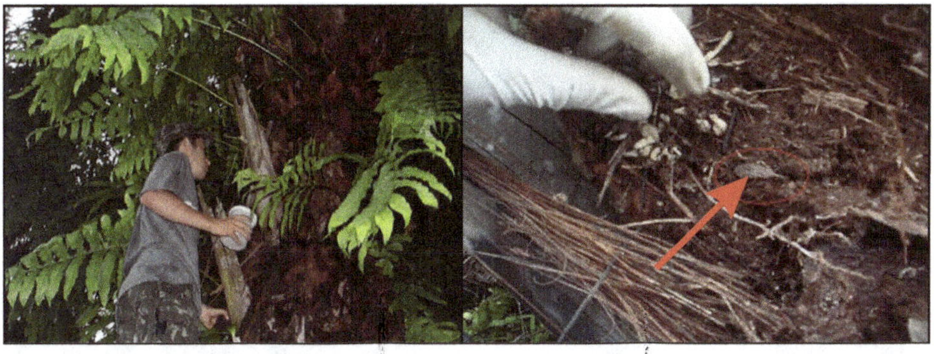

The author setting up traps to collect assassin bugs for epidemiological studies and tropical disease research in the Amazon. This fieldwork took place in January 2000, in the district of Calama, Porto Velho municipality, Rondônia, Brazil.

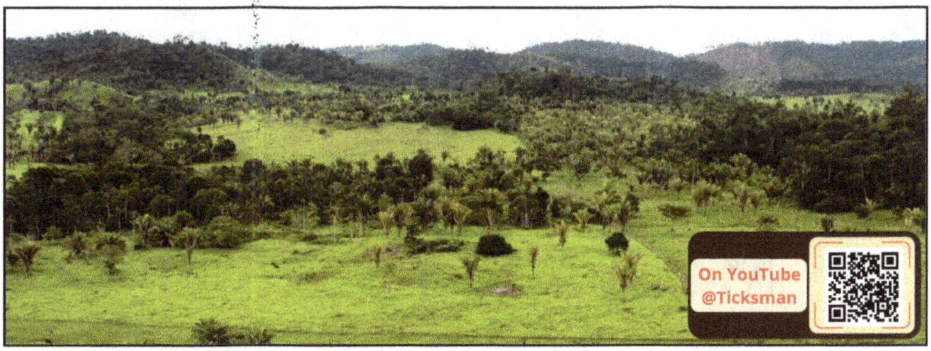

Photo taken in the rural area of Monte Negro, Rondônia. Notice the large number of babassu palm trees, which are abundant in pastures throughout the region and often serve as shelter for assassin bugs (kissing bugs), the vectors of Chagas disease.

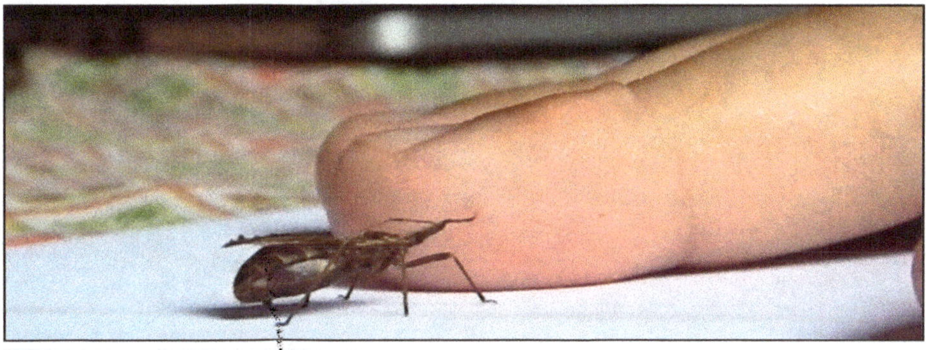

Caught in the act—an assassin bug feeding on a person's finger. Important note: the infective forms of *Trypanosoma cruzi*, the parasite that causes Chagas disease, are released through the insect's feces, not its bite.

Chapter 5

Mechanical Vectors

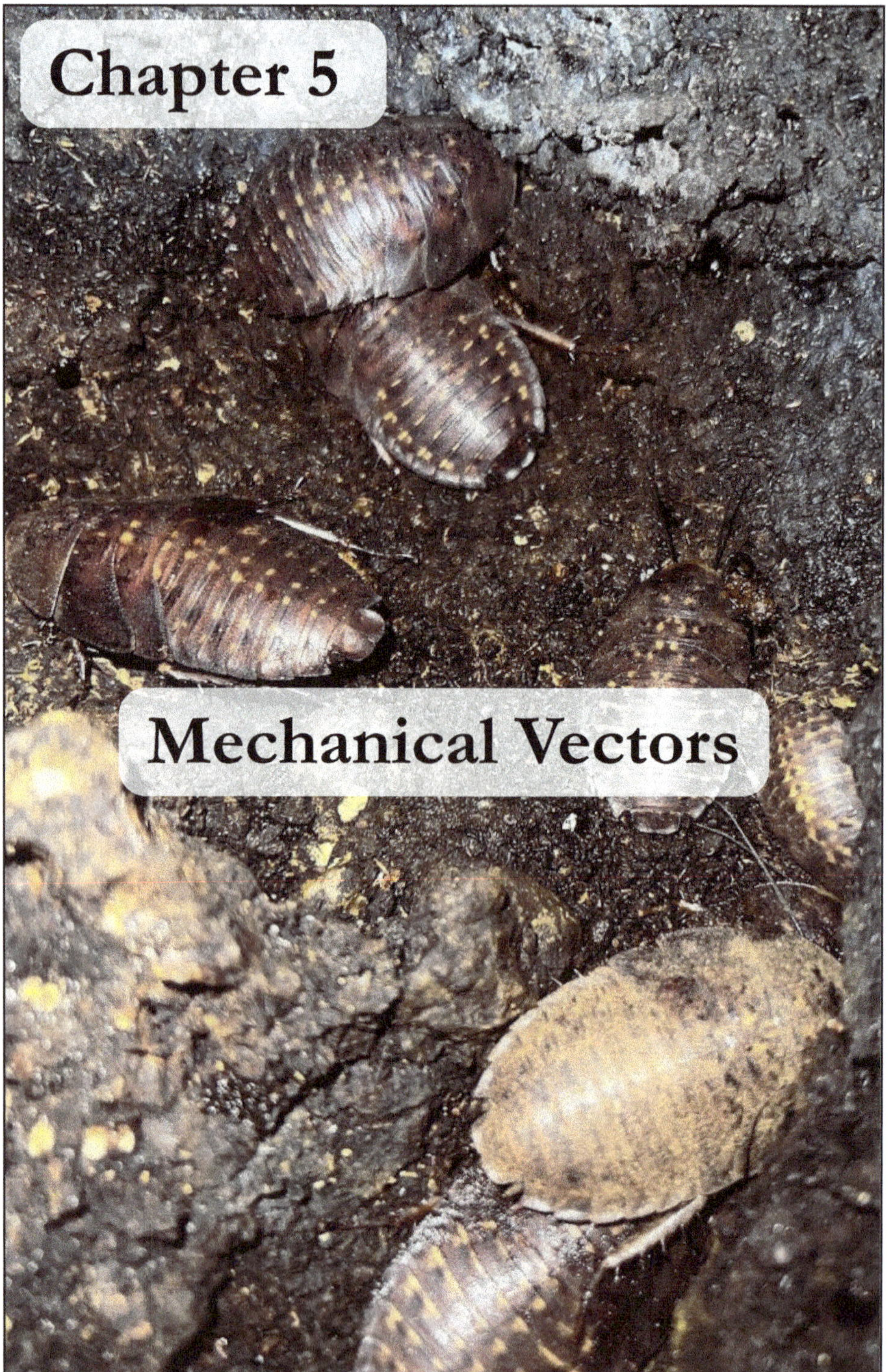

The Invisible Couriers of Microbes

Not every insect needs a bite to bring trouble.

Some just walk across your sandwich, crawl through your toothbrush, or land in your juice... and that's more than enough.

These silent spreaders are called mechanical vectors.
Unlike mosquitoes or ticks—who inject pathogens through bites—mechanical vectors are external transporters. They don't get infected, but they carry microorganisms like bacteria, viruses, fungi, protozoa, and even worm eggs on their feet, legs, antennae, and bodies.

They're the microbial delivery trucks of the insect world—just smaller, faster, and way less welcome.

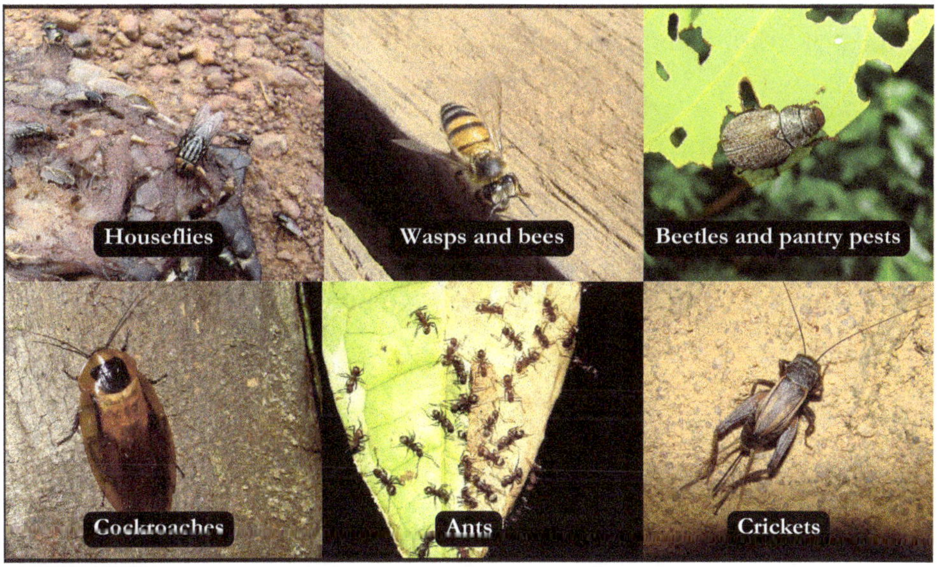

Insects with the potential to carry pathogens on their bodies, legs, or antennae can easily enter our homes and contaminate food, utensils, plates, cups—even our phones. Their presence poses a silent threat to daily hygiene and health.

How Do They Spread Disease?

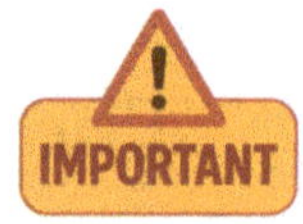

Mechanical vectors become dangerous after contacting:

- Rotting food
- Garbage
- Feces
- Sewage
- Contaminated wounds or medical waste

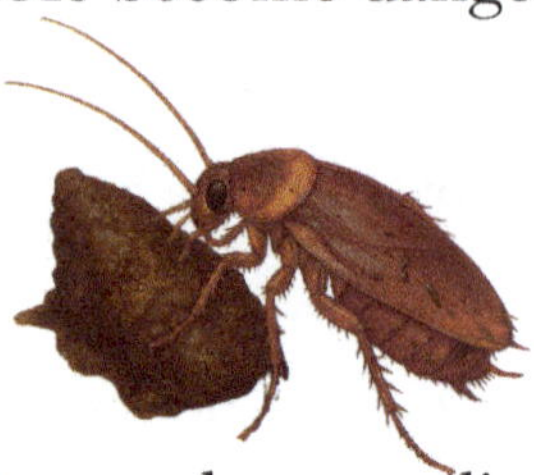

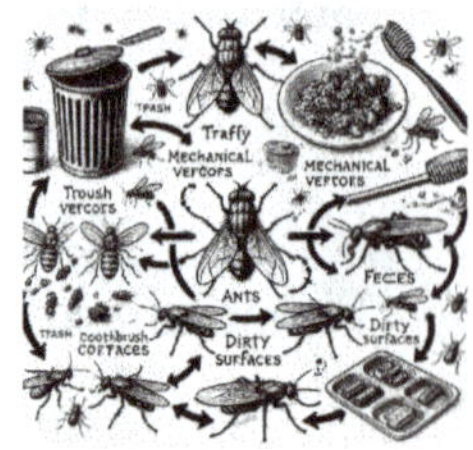

From there, they stroll across:

- Your kitchen counter
- Your school lunch
- Your toothbrush
- Or even hospital beds and instruments

On YouTube
@Ticksman

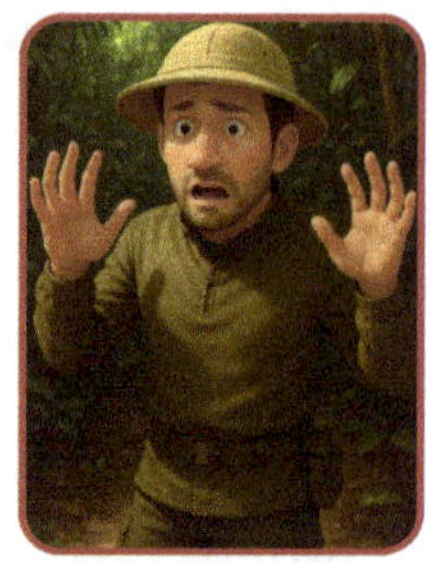

Without even noticing, we can ingest or absorb entire armies of microbes just by touching the same surfaces.

Who Are the Main Culprits?

Some of the most common mechanical vectors include:

- Houseflies – the airborne wanderers of waste and food.
- Cockroaches – sewer-dwelling survivors that love the night shift.
- Ants – sneaky invaders of homes, hospitals, and sugar bowls.
- Pantry beetles and flour moths – invisible until you open the rice.
- Occasional travelers like bees or wasps – rare, but possible microbial messengers.

Each of these insects carries a unique microbial trail, depending on where they've been and what they've walked through.

Why It Matters

Mechanical vectors can:

- Contaminate food, water, and kitchen tools
- Spread intestinal parasites and infectious bacteria
- Trigger allergic reactions and skin infections
- Survive in hidden corners where sprays can't reach
- Thrive in moist, cluttered, and food-rich environments

Even in hospitals, outbreaks of dangerous infections have been traced back to common insects acting as microbial taxis.

What Can We Do?

Prevention is your best defense—and it's easier than you think:

- Keep all food sealed or covered
- Clean up crumbs and spills immediately
- Take out the trash daily and keep bins closed
- Fix any leaky pipes or moisture build-up
- Block entry points with screens and seal cracks
- Use insect baits, sticky traps, or natural repellents
- In shared or public spaces: keep hygiene top-notch

Curious Thought

Mechanical vectors don't mean to harm—they're just doing their insect thing.

But when their "thing" involves walking from poop to your pizza, it's time to act.

So next time you see a bug on your kitchen table…

Ask yourself: "Where have those feet been?"

Knowledge, observation, and a clean space—that's the winning combo to keep these tiny troublemakers away!

In the next sections, we'll explore each of these mechanical vectors in more detail—how they live, what they carry, and most importantly, how we can keep them out of our homes, schools, and kitchens.

Because knowledge is not just power—it's prevention!

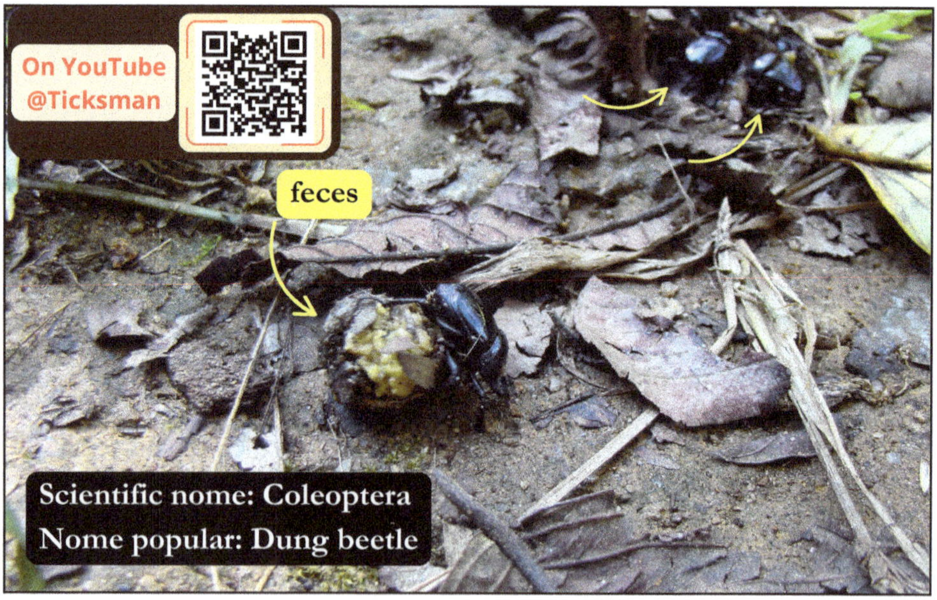
On YouTube
@Ticksman
feces
Scientific nome: Coleoptera
Nome popular: Dung beetle

This image shows a well-known dung beetle rolling cow feces—an important part of its natural behavior. In the background, two others are fighting over a piece of dung. While it's rare for one of these beetles to fly into our homes and land on our food, imagine if it did—what might it bring on its legs besides animal or even human feces? A powerful reminder of how nature's recyclers, though vital in the wild, can pose health risks when crossing into our living spaces.

Cockroaches:
Ancient Crawlers, Modern Threats

They skitter. They hide.

They show up when the lights go off—and they bring along more than just a scare.

Cockroaches are some of the oldest creatures on Earth. They existed even before the dinosaurs and have survived for over 300 million years thanks to their incredible adaptability.

But these ancient survivors are not just harmless bugs—they are powerful mechanical vectors that can carry dozens of disease-causing agents into our homes, hospitals, and food storage areas.

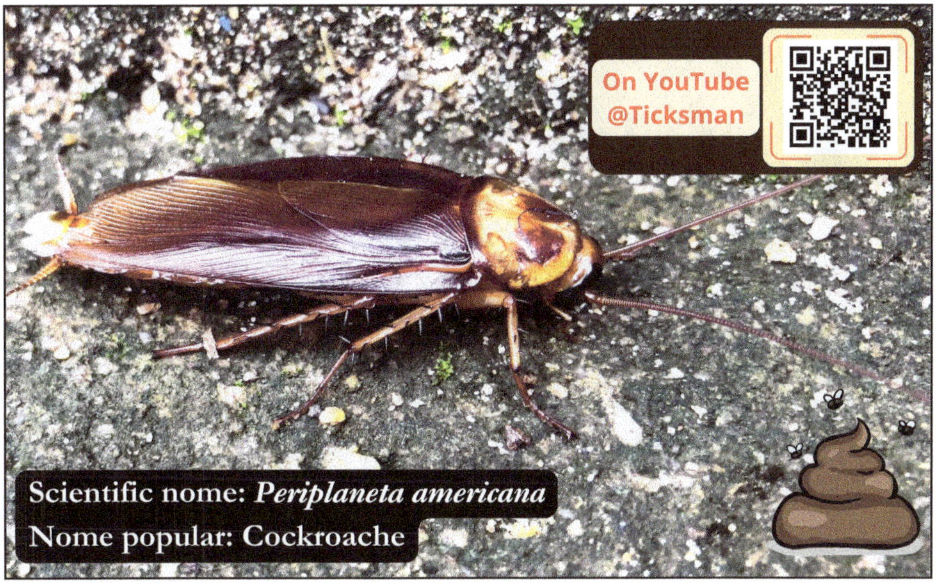

Here we see the infamous red cockroach—*Periplaneta americana*—a true survivor of the insect world. It can live for nearly 30 days without its head and is famously resilient to radiation, even surviving nuclear fallout. But despite all that... there's one thing it can't handle: a flip-flop aimed with precision!

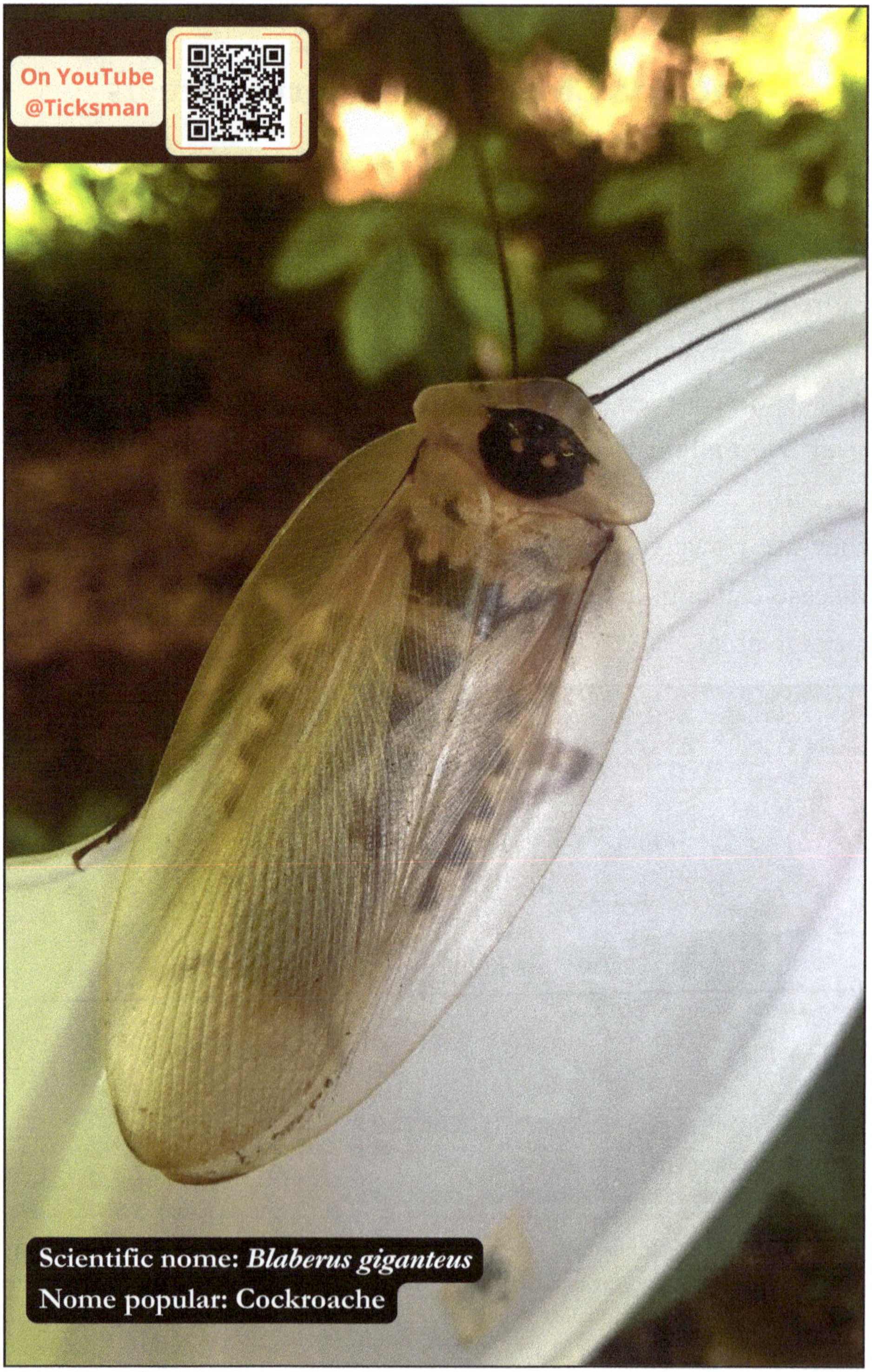
On YouTube
@Ticksman
Scientific nome: *Blaberus giganteus*
Nome popular: Cockroache

What Do Cockroaches Carry?

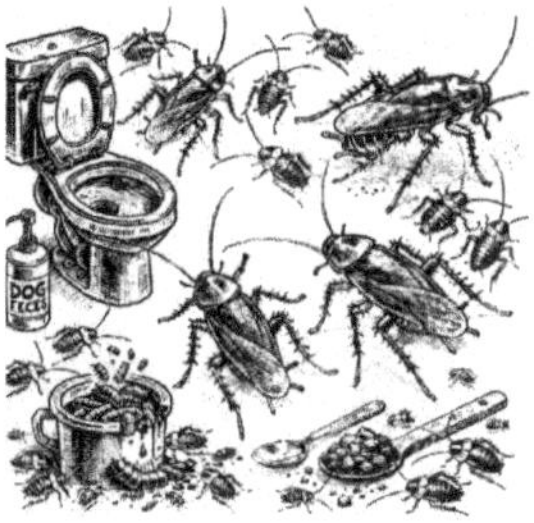

As they crawl through:

- Human and animal feces
- Decaying food and dead animals
- Contaminated hospital waste
- Open wounds, skin flakes, and bodily fluids

They collect a terrifying cargo of bacteria, viruses, fungi, parasite eggs, and protozoa on their legs, antennae, and bodies.

Common diseases linked to cockroaches include:

- Salmonellosis
- *Escherichia coli* infections
- Listeriosis
- Fungal skin infections
- Asthma and allergies (from their feces and body fragments)

The Trouble With Cockroaches

- They are nocturnal – active mostly at night, when we're asleep.
- They love our food – especially open trash cans, crumbs, and dirty dishes.
- They avoid light – their name comes from Latin "blatta", meaning "one that shuns light".
- They reproduce quickly – one female can produce hundreds of offspring.
- They are tough – resistant to many insecticides and can survive without food for weeks.

How to Control Cockroaches: A Global Strategy

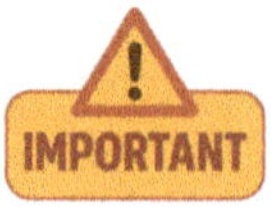

1. Use Baits Wisely

- Pheromone-based traps attract and eliminate male cockroaches, weakening the colony's reproduction.
- Gel baits with poison are placed in corners, cracks, or near sinks.
- **Caution:** If you have pets or small children, place baits in secure areas only!

2. Control at Night

- Clean thoroughly before bedtime.
- Empty trash cans, clean counters, and seal food containers.
- Baratas love the night shift—cut off their buffet!

3. Seal Entry Points

- Close cracks in walls, baseboards, and windows.
- Fix leaks and eliminate moisture—cockroaches love damp areas.

4. Keep It Clean

- Don't leave dirty dishes overnight.
- Vacuum crumbs under stoves, refrigerators, and furniture.
- Clean food storage areas regularly.

5. Natural Options (with Caution)

- Some cultures use bay leaves, cucumber peels, or boric acid —but these have mixed results.
- Diatomaceous earth (a natural powder) can dry out their exoskeletons—safe for humans and pets if used correctly.

6. Call the Experts

- If the infestation is large, contact professional pest control.
- They may use foggers, sprays, or fumigation based on severity.

Fun Fact

Cockroaches can survive for up to a week without their head and hold their breath for 40 minutes!

That's why it takes more than a quick spray to truly get rid of them.

Final Tip for Parasite Hunters

Cockroaches are more than just creepy—they are tiny, crawling disease dispensers.

By keeping your home clean, food sealed, and baits well-placed, you become the ultimate guardian against one of the world's oldest pests.

Don't let them win the night. 🌙🪳🚫

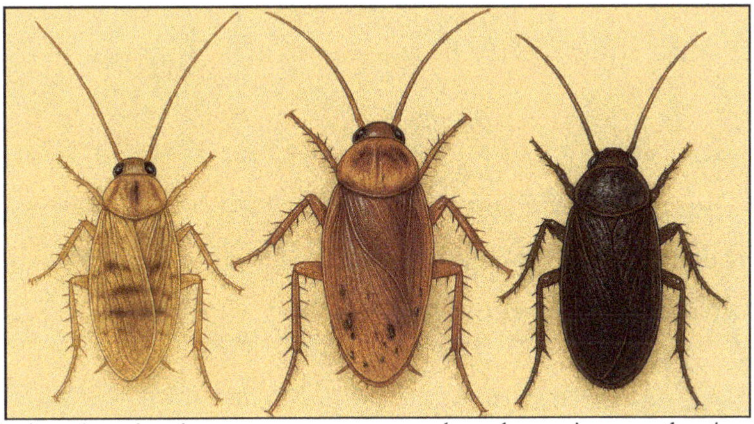

In South America, the three most common cockroach species are: the tiny German cockroach (*Blattella germanica*), also known locally as the "francesinha"; the larger American cockroach (*Periplaneta americana*), often found near sewage; and the shiny dark Oriental cockroach (*Blatta orientalis*). All of them love to stay close to our food—so beware!

Ants: Tiny Invaders in Homes and Hospitals

Ants may look harmless, but they can be dangerous transporters of microbes.

In hospitals, ants have been found carrying:

- Bacteria like *Staphylococcus* and *Pseudomonas*
- Fungal spores
- Pathogens from wounds, medical waste, or contaminated equipment

At home, ants travel between trash, toilets, pet food, and our kitchens, spreading bacteria on legs and antennae.

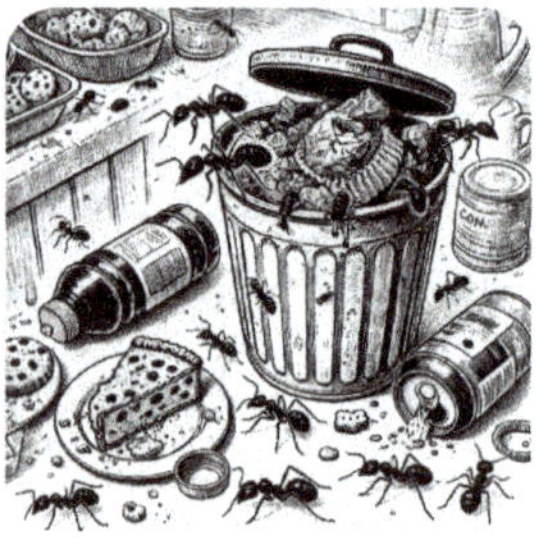

Control Tips:

- Seal cracks and food containers.
- Clean up spills and crumbs immediately.
- Avoid leaving pet food out overnight.
- Use safe indoor ant baits—keep away from children and pets.

Houseflies: Wings That Spread Disease

Houseflies don't bite—but they are one of the most notorious mechanical vectors in the world.

They land on:

- Feces, garbage, and dead animals
- Then crawl over our food, utensils, and hands

They carry over 100 pathogens, including:

- *Salmonella*
- *E. coli*
- Cholera and typhoid bacteria
- Parasitic eggs and viruses

Control Tips:

- Keep windows and doors screened.
- Cover all food—especially in outdoor areas.
- Dispose of garbage daily and keep lids closed.
- Clean drains and kitchen surfaces regularly.

Topic: Other Arthropods in Our Homes – Bees, Beetles, Crickets & More

Not all arthropods that enter our homes are harmful, but they can still carry parasites or pathogens much like cockroaches, houseflies, and ants. In this book, we won't dive deeply into groups like bees, beetles, or crickets. However, it's important to know:

Bees play a crucial role in pollination, helping produce much of the food we eat. Despite their ecological importance, they are venomous—multiple stings can be dangerous, even fatal for some people.

As for other insects, if you notice an unusual number of them indoors or around your home, especially if it's sudden or excessive, call a pest control specialist. Stay alert and remember: awareness is prevention. But don't worry—these fascinating creatures are a story for another book!

The Parasite Hunt:
A Challenge for the Brave!

Are you ready to uncover the secrets of the hidden world of parasites? This book is not just a journey into the microscopic universe—it's an adventure! Throughout its pages, you will find mysteries, codes, and hidden clues leading you deeper into the world of tropical parasites.

Your mission? Decipher the challenges and reach the final prize!

How It Works:

✔ The game begins with the first hidden clue inside this book.
✔ Each clue leads to the next step, revealing the path to the ultimate mystery.
✔ You'll need to decode texts, use maps, and scan QR Codes to progress.
✔ The final challenge will unlock a special VIP Group where you'll have direct access to the author for more exclusive adventures and discussions!

Hint: The first key lies in the dedication. What do the numbers reveal? Ready?

🏆 The Prizes!

🎁 Grand Prize: Unlock the final QR Code and join the VIP Group of The Parasite Hunters, where you can:

Chat directly with the author about tropical parasites and Amazonian adventures.

Receive exclusive challenges and bonus content.

Be the first to hear about future books, events, and discoveries.

🎁 Bonus Rewards: Some milestones along the way may unlock surprise gifts, from secret parasite facts to exclusive downloadable content.

🧩 Ready for the Hunt?

The first step awaits! Look carefully, think critically, and trust your instincts—just like a true parasite tracker in the wild. Scan, decode, and explore!

1	2	3	4	5	6	7	8	9	10	11	12	13	14	15	16	17	18	19	20	21	22	23	24	25	26
a	**b**	**c**	**d**	**e**	**f**	**g**	**h**	**i**	**j**	**k**	**l**	**m**	**n**	**o**	**p**	**q**	**r**	**s**	**t**	**u**	**v**	**x**	**w**	**y**	**z**

1. **How many Qr-codes are there in the TikTok book?** [*First letter*]
2. **How many Qr-codes are there in the YouTube book?** [*second and third letters*]
3. **Where is the female mosquito (*Anopheles darlingi*) biting the author's foot?** *Find the photo in the book. The page number is the letter you're missing!*

Keep hunting, Parasite Hunter! 🕵️📓🕷️

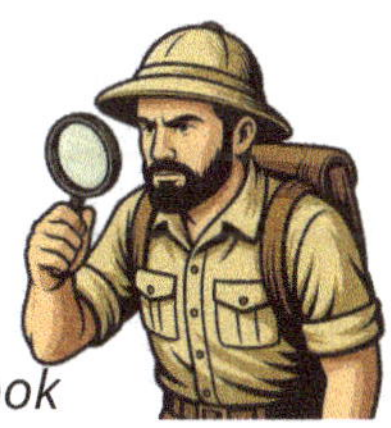

Scan the QR-Code where this animal is in the book

About the Author

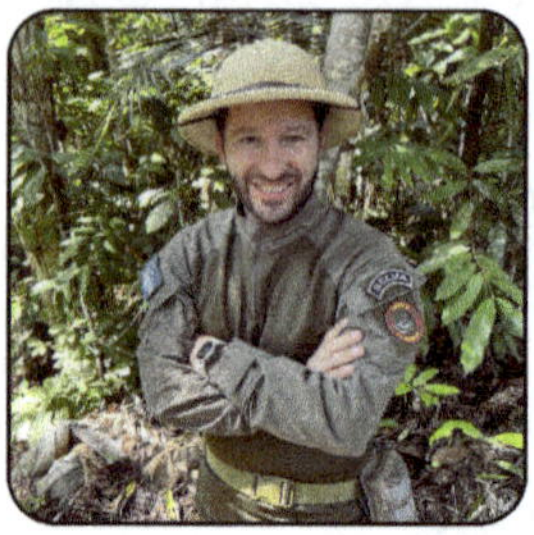

Flávio Aparecido Terassini is a passionate Brazilian biologist, parasitologist, tropical disease researcher, university professor, and science communicator who has studied parasitology and tropical diseases in the Amazon since 1999. He has dedicated his life to the biodiversity of the rainforest and has discovered numerous new species of arthropods. Flávio holds a degree in Biology (2005) and a Master's in Pathogen-Host Biology from the prestigious University of São Paulo (USP, 2011), and he is currently a PhD candidate at the Bionorte Network (2023). He has been a university professor of Medicine since 2006 and has served as the Coordinator of Biology and Agronomy at UniSL, where he also leads innovation and employability initiatives. Throughout his career, he has collaborated with USP's ICB5, Instituto Butantan, Brazil's Ministry of Health, Cemetron Infectious Disease Hospital, and the Brazilian Armed Forces. He has authored four published books and one book chapter, published over 27 scientific papers in national and international journals, and presented more than 39 papers at scientific congresses. From 2017 to 2023, he was a radio columnist for CBN Amazônia 101.9 FM, and he has been a consultant for Rede Amazônica (Globo) since 2004 and a featured guest on AmazonSat TV since 2019. He is also the founder and CEO of Terassini – Courses, Lectures & Consultancies, and the creator of the scientific YouTube channel and TikTok: Ticksman, where he shares real-life adventures with parasites and insights from the Amazon. Through this book, he invites readers not only to learn, but to explore, play, and protect the living world of the invisible creatures that surround us.

References and Further Reading

Barros-Battesti DM, Arzua M, Bechara GH. **Carrapatos de importância médico-veterinária da região neotropical: um guia ilustrado para identificação de espécies.** São Paulo: Vox/ICTTD-3/Butantan; 2006.

Galvão C, editor. **Vetores da Doença de Chagas no Brasil.** 1st ed. São Paulo: Sociedade Brasileira de Zoologia; 2014.

Hanson PE, Nishida K. **Insects and other arthropods of tropical America.** 1st ed. Ithaca (NY): Cornell University Press; 2016.

Linardi PM, Guimarães LR. **Sifonápteros do Brasil.** 1st ed. São Paulo: Museu de Zoologia da Universidade de São Paulo; 2000.

Nava S, Venzal JM, González-Acuña D, Martins TF, Guglielmone AA. **Ticks of the Southern Cone of America: Diagnosis, Distribution, and Hosts with Taxonomy, Ecology and Sanitary Importance.** 1st ed. London: Academic Press; 2017.

Rey L. **Bases da parasitologia médica.** 3rd ed. Rio de Janeiro: Guanabara Koogan; 2010.

Rey L. **Parasitologia: parasitos e doenças parasitárias do homem nas Américas e na África.** 3rd ed. Rio de Janeiro: Guanabara Koogan; 2001.

Terassini FA. **Amazon Rainforest Secrets.** Kindle ed. 1st ed. Amazon. Chicago, EUA; 2020.

Terassini FA. **Histórias Arrepiantes de João Biologão sobre os Parasitas.** Kindle ed. 1st ed. Amazon; Chicago, EUA. 2020.

Terassini FA. **Guia Completo de Artrópodes Peçonhentos.** Kindle ed. Amazon; v.2. Chicago, EUA, 2021.

www.ingramcontent.com/pod-product-compliance
Lightning Source LLC
Chambersburg PA
CBHW061214240926
51846CB00006B/1220